COMPREHENSIVE STUDY
OF ICD-10
DIAGNOSTIC MEDICAL CODING
FOR PHYSICIANS
AND OUTPATIENT SERVICES

By Dr. Lyn Olsen
RHIT, CCS, CPC-H, CCS-P, CPC

This book is dedicated to the extraordinary women of my family who always inspired everyone to be their best – this includes my mother Myrna Mae Miller and her sisters Alice and Donna, and their mom Lilian, with the greatness continuing on in my sister Rebecca and cousin Devvi and my daughters, Teressa Lyn and Gemavie Marie.

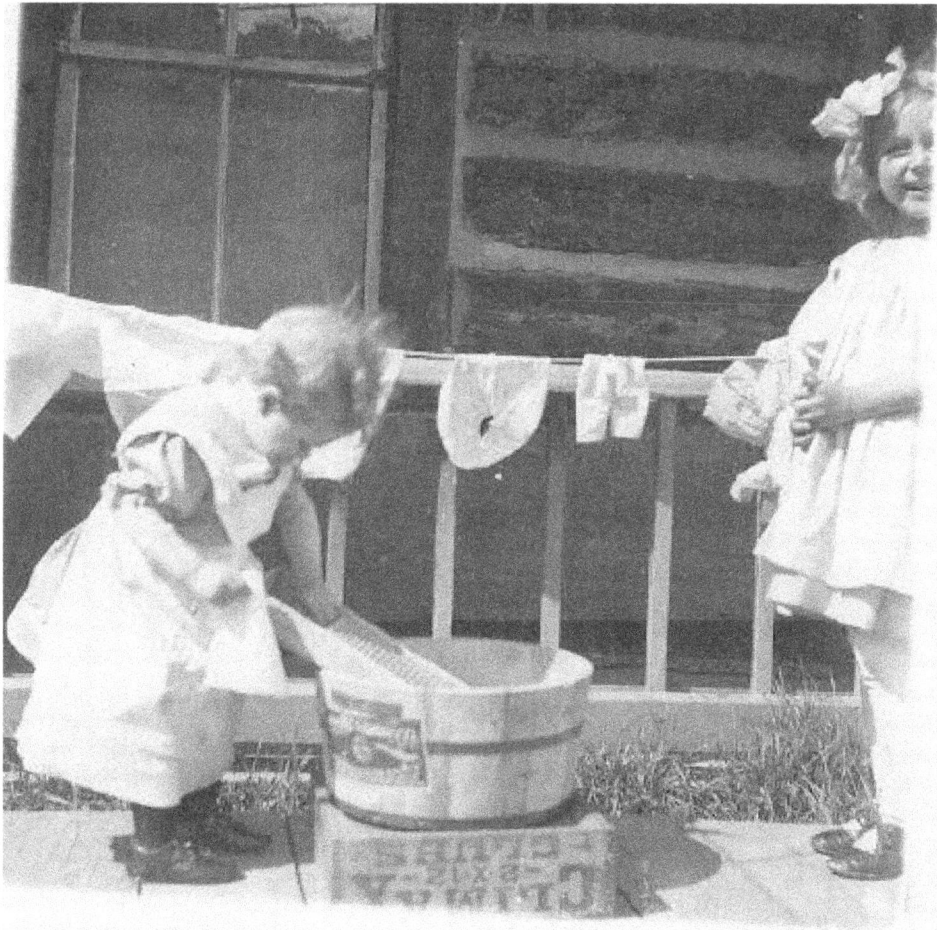

TABLE OF CONTENTS

CHAPTER 1

HEALTH ADMINISTRATION

You will learn the following objectives in this chapter:

A. Knowledge of the beginning and development of the health administration field.
B. Definition and history of a hierarchial system.
C. Knowledge of the history and development of ICD-10-CM.
D. Define terminology used for understanding ICD-10-CM.
E. Current role and application of coding within health administration.

Section 1.1: HISTORY OF MEDICAL CODING

One of the primary systems used in medical coding is the International Classification of Diseases (ICD). The origin of this concept dates back to the ancient civilizations for the purpose of tracking and classifying diseases and causes of illnesses and death which have always intrigued mankind, but also has the purpose of promoting better health and eliminating causes of death. Today, ICD is the world's most widely used classification system.

More recently, in the 17th century, the English statistician, John Graunt, developed the London Bills of Mortality which identified the number of children who died before reaching age 6 and mimicked the same basis of earlier disease and death classification systems. Later in 1838, William Farr, registrar general of England, developed a system to classify deaths.

It was the Bertillon Classification of Causes of Death, however, that was developed in 1893 that became the precursor for the ICD system. This was developed by a French physician, Jacques Bertillon at the International Statistical Institute in Chicago. Subsequently, in 1898 the American Public Health Association (APHA) recommended the adoption of the Bertillon System with revisions every ten years. In 1900 the first international conference was convened to revise what now is known as the International Classification of Causes of Death.

The Mixed Commission, a group composed of representatives from the International Statistical Institute and the Health Organization of the League of Nations, was responsible for the early revisions. Early revisions contained minor changes, but there were major changes in the sixth revision when it changed from one book to two books (known as tabular and alphabetical volumes) as well as changing of the title to Manual of International Statistical Classification of Diseases, Injuries and Causes of Death (ICD). Ever since there have been numerous revisions which are a reflection of the changes in healthcare, diseases, and knowledge within the health field.

Section 1.2: DEVELOPMENT OF ICD

It was in 1948 that the World Health Organization (WHO), headquartered in Geneva, Switzerland, assumed responsibility for the revisions of the ICD with the production of the 7th version in 1957 and the eighth revision in 1968. WHO designed ICD for classification of morbidity and mortality information for statistical purposes and for indexing medical records by disease and operations.

It was in 1968 that the Eighth Revision of International Classification of Diseases (ICD) was published in the United States and served as the basis for coding diagnostic data for official morbidity and mortality statistics in the U.S. When revised by United States, ICD was modified and utilized for purposes of billing, thus this version became known as the Clinical Modification (CM); therefore, this revision became known as ICD-8-CM.

The purpose of the book has remained to encompass the great variety and complexity, as well as technological advances in healthcare, in the diagnosis and treatment of diseases and other conditions that influence a person's well-being. It was able to emphasize what was happening clinically; namely, to serve as a useful tool in the area of classification of morbidity data for identification of diagnoses, demonstrating medical necessity, indexing of medical records, medical review, ambulatory and other medical care programs, as well as for basic health statistics. This version of the ICD then expanded to a third volume to be used by hospitals for coding procedures and introduced the fifth character subclassification.

Section 1.3: UPDATES TO ICD

Regardless of the version of the ICD, there are updates added October 1st of every year with clarifications and explanations provided routinely which can be accessed through the government's Federal Register. Updates are issued periodically by what is now known as the Centers for Medicare and Medicaid Services (CMS) or formerly known as the Health Care Financing Administration (HCFA). CMS is a part of the United States Federal Government's Health and Human Services Department.

The most current revision ICD-10 has been released by WHO but has not been adopted by the United States due to the many changes that need to be made so that the codes can be used for various other purposes including reimbursement as well as the need for coordination between the many agencies and associations involved in the use of the codes. The four primary agencies responsible for updates in United States are American Hospital Association (AHA), National Center for Health Statistics (NCHS), American Health Information Management Association (AHIMA), and Centers for Medicare and Medicaid Services (CMS). Other agencies involved in updating the ICD are American Association of Health Data Systems, American Academy of Pediatrics, American College of Physicians, American College of Surgeons, American Medical Association (AMA), and WHO Center for Classification of Diseases.

Section 1.4: NATIONAL CODING ORGANIZATIONS

There are two national organizations recognized for national certification of medical coders which is the American Health Information Management Association (AHIMA) and American Academic of Professional Coders (AAPC).

AMERICAN HEALTH INFORMATION MANAGEMENT ASSOCIATION (AHIMA):
AHIMA is a well known health administration national organization that has been in existence for over 75 years. It was formed in 1928 by the Association of Record Librarians to standardize

and professionalize the health care administration field. Currently there are over 70,000 registered members and many more professionals who have been certified through the various certifications offered by AHIMA. AHIMA is headquartered in Chicago, Illinois. The organization provides a wide variety of other services besides certification which includes development of standards and government regulations, seminars, training, accreditation, publications, and continuing education.

While a person may gain certification, they do not necessarily have to be members although additional benefits are provided to members such as lower costs for tests, publications, and conferences in addition to access to information and publications. Membership costs are reduced for students who are attending an accredited AHIMA school. AHIMA offers an immense variety of publications, including textbooks and sample certification tests.

Various certifications through AHIMA include Registered Health Information Technicians (RHITs) and Registered Health Information Administrators (RHIAs). These national certifications are often required for various administrative positions within hospitals or large clinics. In addition, AHIMA now offers certifications for management of privacy and security programs within medical practices. These certifications are known as Certified in Healthcare Privacy (CHP) and Certified in Healthcare Security (CHS); a combined certification, can be obtained.

AHIMA provides coding certification for both physician (Certified Coding -Specialist–Physician Based, CCS-P) and hospital (Certified Coding Specialist, CCS for inpatient and outpatient hospital coding). In addition, there is certification for entry-level coders (Certified Coding Associate, CCA). It is also recommended that you have several years' experience within the coding and billing fields before taking the CCS-P and CCS exams.

AHIMA can be contacted at their website (www.ahima.org), where applications, forms, and information are provided. In addition, this website provides sample tests, description of available references, listing of AHIMA-certified educational resources, correspondence material, and various other coding-related information. Materials can be purchased for a home study course in coding, but not for RHIT or RHIA which requires an associates or bachelor's degree from an AHIMA accredited school.

AMERICAN ACADEMY OF PROFESSIONAL CODERS (AAPC): The American Academy of Professional Coders (AAPC) was formed in 1988 and provides national coding certification for both physician (Certified -Professional Coder, CPC) and hospital (Certified Outpatient Coder, COC and Certified Inpatient Coder, CIC). They also offer certification in auditing, management, and compliance. AAPC is composed of a national advisory board with members selected from state organizations. AAPC is supported by a national physician advisory board. There are now more than 150,000 members throughout 250 local chapters. There are state and local groups that provide educational opportunities and meetings for its members.

AAPC can be contacted at their website (www.aapc.com), where form, dates, application, and information are provided. In addition, this website provides sample tests, description of available references, listing of AAPC-certified educational resources, correspondence material, and various other coding-related information. Coursework can be purchased for a home study course. Dates are also available in AAPC's publication, "The Coding Edge," or by calling the national office. Locations and dates of exams are determined by local AAPC chapters.

CHAPTER 2
REGULATIONS AND COMPLIANCE

You will learn the following objectives in this chapter:

A. Definitions of fraud and abuse.
B. Report Formats
C. Types of Health Record Formats
D. Types of Reports
E. Patient Records
F. Healthcare Quality
G. Legislation pertinent to fraud and abuse.
H. Agencies involved in fraud and abuse prosecution.
I. Elements of a compliance program.
J. OIG Workplan
K. Auditing

Section 2.1: TYPES OF OFFENSES

There are three levels at which healthcare offenses can occur. Fraud is the most severe offense as it is considered the purposeful intent to gain funds from the rendering of healthcare in an illegal manner. Abuse is based on the failure to perform fair and reasonable billing and coding practices as illustrated by the standardized practices throughout other healthcare providers. The least offensive are acts of omission and mistakes since they are supposed to not contain any purposeful intent to defraud. The classification of these errors are evaluated based on the practices of the healthcare provider, so if a provider is attempting in good faith to comply with the rules and regulations and has instituted standard practices and procedures, then errors would most likely be considered to be actions of omissions and mistakes.

The importance of fraud and abuse concepts within a healthcare practice are critical and fearsome to healthcare providers. The government estimates that billions of dollars are lost every year to healthcare fraud and abuse. Providers who act properly should not have to worry, however, as qualified personnel who are knowledgeable and up-to-date on rules and regulations can ensure that proper procedures are instituted to protect the practice and to ensure proper reimbursement. One important aspect of a certified coder or health administration would be the institution of a compliance program to ensure proper controls and procedures are instituted to assure compliance with federal rules and regulations, as well as state and local.

While computerized programs are utilized to create profiles of healthcare practices, these are used to determine inconsistencies or poor practices and which may trigger federal audits. Examples of fraud or abuse can include:
   (1)   Upcoding means the selection of codes at a higher level than as justified by the documentation within the patient's record.
   (2)   Downcoding means the selection of codes at a lower level than as justified by the documentation with the patient's record.
   (3)   Billing for noncovered services using codes for covered services.

(4)   Billing for services provided that were not medically necessary.
(5)   Misuse of modifiers.
(6)   Misuse of place of service on the billing form.
(7)   Using ICD-10 codes to justify billing when the patient does not have the diagnosis.
(8)   Altering claims fraudulently after they have already been submitted in order to increase payment.
(9)   Billings for services not rendered.
(10)   Billing for office visits when only surgical procedures were performed.
(11)   Unbundling of global services.
(12)   Overutilization and billing of laboratory or radiological services.
(13)   Billing for consultations when an office visit was provided.
(14)   Improper billing for physician services when services are provided by other staff who are not qualified to provide the service for billing purposes.
(15)   Billing for services by two physicians for a surgical procedure that is not billable as a team procedure.
(16)   Changing of dates of service to ensure additional payments.
(17)   Duplicate billing.
(18)   Billing and/or performing a more costly procedure, lab, or test when not justified as medically necessary.
(19)   Misidentifying the person receiving the services for billing purposes.
(20)   Kickbacks, bribes, rebates or other remuneration in exchange for services and referrals.
(21)   Routine waivers of copays and deductibles which can be construed to be an inducement to gain referrals and patients.

Section 2.2: REPORT FORMATS

There are a number of important policies/procedures and data that must be followed and provided to ensure standardization on the medical record to reduce any misinterpretations since records may be shared amongst different medical specialties and across the country or nations.

As part of the effort to standardize health record data, the Uniform Hospital and Discharge Data Set (UHDDS) was established. UHDDS required that certain information be included in all medical records across the country which includes: patient full name, patient identifier number, address, date of birth, gender, marital status, race or ethnic group, social security number, primary and secondary insurance companies and information, guarantor for patient's account, employer's name and address, parent information for minor child, occupation, emergency contact information, primary care physician contact information and referring physician. This ensures that if a patient moves to another part of the country they can still receive optimal healthcare in that it is not jeopardized by a lack of communication or information.

Other data sets collect similar data as well as additional data relative to the type of care. These include the Minimum Data Set for Long-Term Care (MDS) used for nursing home patients, the Uniform Ambulatory Care Data Set (UACDS) for ambulatory patients, the Outcomes and Assessment Information Set (OASIS) for home health patients, Data Elements for Emergency

Department Systems (DEEDS) for emergency room patients, and Health Plan Employer Data and Information Set (HEDIS) for healthcare purchasers and patients.

Section 2.3: TYPES OF HEALTH RECORD FORMATS

There are three main types of health record formats: source oriented, integrated, and problem oriented.

A source-oriented health record is based on what department, specialty, or other group is involved in the patient's care. This type of report makes it easy to find and follow specific treatment of a patient. For instance, all of the x-rays for a patient diagnosed with cancer would be located together and it would be easy to follow the progression of the disease. The problem, though, is that it can result in fragmentation of the history of care as other specialties may provide services pertinent to other services which results in a less congruent time frame of care. It is also dependent on the knowledge of what kind of records and care is being sought before reports can be located which may result in some information being overlooked.

An integrated health record is where all reports are strictly situated within the record chronologically. Although this may provide a more congruent time line for the patient's care, this can be highly cumbersome, particularly for lengthy files in which there may be many reports. In this type of format, each report would be viewed in order to progress to the next one until the desired report is found.

A problem-oriented health record is based on the diagnosis or problem for which the patient is being treated. This type of format is also known as POMR (problem oriented medical record). This format presents the difficulty of comprehending the patient's record of care if a patient has numerous problems and many services are provided.

An alternative to these three types of health record formats include a format which combines various aspects of each format which can be selected and implemented according to the needs of the healthcare practice.

Progress notes are used often by healthcare providers and may be presented in several formats. The SOAP is the most common format consisting of four categories. This consists of the description of each category sometimes contained within a couple of sentences in the order of SOAP. The S stands for subjective which is the symptoms and history as stated by the patient and usually obtained from the health history record completed by the patient prior to services being provided. The O stands for objective which is the findings of the healthcare provider. A stands for Assessment which is the evaluation and determination by the healthcare provider of the patient's condition. The P stand for plan which is the healthcare provider's decision regarding what type of care will be provided to the patient. This format is enhanced in the SNOCAMP format. The additional elements are N which means nature of presenting problem, C which means counseling and/or coordination of care, and M which means medical decision making.

Section 2.4: TYPES OF REPORTS

There are numerous reports that can be found within a medical record. The main ones for hospitalization include History and Physical, Operative, Consultations, Pathology, Radiology, and Discharge Summary. Offices frequently use progress notes as previously described, but the other report types will be described here.

It is important to understand medical record formats as a coder because documentation is where the codes are derived from during asbstracting. Abstracting is the higher level process in which coders take the entire medical record with all reports and research through them to find the ICD-9 diagnostic codes and CPT/HCPCS codes in physician billing. With hospital coding, Volume 3 ICD-10-PCS procedural codes would be used instead of CPT codes. As a coder, you will have to read and review the many reports found within the record and, therefore, the more familiar you are with the record format and what is contained within the reports, the easier it will be to find the right information to ensure proper coding.

The best reports have clearly defined headings which include patient information at the beginning followed by specific headings relative to the report which will be discussed for each report. As a coder, you will use these headings to help you scan a record and know where important information is located and where your analysis as a coder should begin and what it should include. When you first begin abstracting from reports you will find it cumbersome and slow but as you progress you will learn where crucial information is located and, therefore, will became faster.

As with all reports, the History and Physical report begins with demographics, such as the patient's name, patient number, physician's name, etc. There is usually an ADMITTING DIAGNOSIS listed. This heading section is then followed by paragraphs. These paragraphs usually begin with a HISTORY OF PRESENT ILLNESS, followed by PAST FAMILY SOCIAL HISTORY, ALLERGIES, and REVIEW OF SYSTEMS. You will learn more about the value of these sections in determining the level of evaluation and management codes with CPT coding later. The paragraphs then progress onto the EXAM, and an IMPRESSION. When these reports are properly done, the REVIEW OF SYSTEMS and EXAM sections will contain subsections highlighted by the different systems of the body, such as HEENT, CARDIOVASCULAR, RESPIRATORY, INTEGUMENTARY, DIGESTIVE, etc.

The Operative Report consists of the regular headings as previously mentioned including a listing of the diagnoses and the operative procedure. It is this brief description of the procedure in this heading that is a critical beginning point for determining what services were provided for CPT coding purposes. The report then proceeds into the paragraph sections which consists primarily of a description of the procedure. Remember as you gain experience you will get faster with abstracting information from the reports.

Pathology reports usually consist of the standard headings in addition to the postoperative diagnoses, specimens, gross description, and microscopic description. Radiology consists of the standard headings in addition to the type of test and the findings.

The last report is typically the Discharge Summary which also contains the standard headings but includes a DISCHARGE DIAGNOSES. It is this heading that is the most important within all of the reports because it is the most definitive diagnoses and is where you should start when you are abstracting. You should use other diagnostic listings and descriptions to verify this or add to it, in addition to various paragraphs throughout the patient's chart. There is usually a description of the hospital stay, a brief description of the procedure, and then a discharge plan.

Section 2.5: PATIENT RECORDS

A personal health record (PHR) contains personal health information (PHI) which if stored electronically is known as electronic health record (EHR).

Minimum required information in the data set for the these can include demographic information, medical information, allergies, conditions, hospitalizations, surgeries, medications, immunizations, provider information, health status, medical, personal and family history, insurances, and payments.

It must be remembered that the PHI is owned by the patient, the PRH is controlled by the patient, but the EHR are property of the healthcare provider. The PHR differs from the EHR in that the patient controls the information in the PHR and maintains it.

There are various methods used with the EHR. This includes voice recognition, bar code readers, computer templates, computerized data entry systems, document imaging, computerized physician order entry (CPOE), and optical character readers.

With an electronic system, there must be a process in which signatures can be authenticated. This means that the computer system can provide electronic signatures by various means which are used to indicate that the person entering the information entered into the electronic record is the authorized person and not somebody else. This can be achieved by the use of passwords, user ID, and other means of identification. It is critical that the person who is authorized with that signature is the one entering the information and that nobody else ever enters information on another person's electronic signature.

Release of information (ROI) is as form that allows the release of patient information to another agency or party. The information provided should follow the minimum necessary standards in which health information should be limited to the minimum amount that will achieve the purpose of the request. Per HIPAA, the information on the ROI should include
- o The patient's name and date of birth
- o Doctor's full name
- o What is being requested and who is requesting
- o Expiration date or event that relates to the individual or the purpose of the use or disclosure
- o Revocable clause
- o AIDS confidentiality clause
- o Signed recently
- o A statement regarding the potential for redisclosure of information

Section 2.6: HEALTHCARE QUALITY

Healthcare quality is overseen by Centers for Medicare and Medicaid Services (CMS) as well as Agency for Healthcare Research and Quality (AHRQ) which is also part of HSS. The National Committee for Quality Assurance (NCQA) also works with promoting quality healthcare. They are responsible for developing the Health Plan Employer Data and Information Set (HEDIS) and are involved in accreditation and certification with the purpose that employers are able to select healthcare plans. The American National Standards Institute (ANSI) provides accreditation to organizations to ensure utilization of proper standards. The American Society for Testing and Materials (ASTM) establishes standards for materials and products.

Section 2.7: LEGISLATION

There are many pieces of legislation that affect healthcare reimbursement and practice, as well as there are many governmental agencies that monitor, deny reimbursement, and prosecute false or inaccurate claims. If a claim is successfully prosecuted, the monies can amount fast due to various aspects of legislation. Fines can include $10,000 per incident in addition to three times the amount of the fraud. Although this may not sound ominous at first, it must be recognized that such an event of fraud and abuse may be found to have occurred in 5% of the files over a number of years, so the fine is computed based on each incident and can easily amount to millions of dollars. Penalties can also include prison time and loss of privileges to serve government patients, such as Medicare patients who may constitute the larger portion of a healthcare practice's business and, therefore, put them out of business. In addition, the government will issue a corporate integrity agreement (CIA) which lists specific restrictions on the operations of the practice to ensure proper compliance and correction of abuse procedures. To view examples, the government's website can be accessed at www.oig.hhs.gov.

Legislation to combat fraud and abuse include the False Claims Act, Stark Laws, anti-kickback laws, Qui Tam actions, Health Insurance Portability and Accountability Act (HIPAA), and the deficit reduction act.

The False Claims Act was designed during the Civil War to address false claims by military contractors but is still actively used today. It prohibits the submission of false claims to the government.

The anti-kickback laws are to prevent fraud and abuse by ensuring that providers do not recommend that their patients receive services from an organization or provider who is affiliated with the initial provider. This includes companies owned by the referring provider or their families or associates or with whom the provider or their family or associates are partners which, therefore results in the referring provider receiving benefits, including monetary or otherwise. These types of kickbacks are addressed under the Stark laws. This also includes the referring of patients by a provider to someone he may not know professionally or personally, but who are giving the provider benefits for the referral. In other words, the provider cannot refer a patient to any entity from which he or she will benefit either monetarily or in any other manner. Kickbacks have occurred with pharmaceutical companies, durable medical equipment companies, and laboratories.

Qui tam means that a private plaintiff files a lawsuit in place of the government.

In the Deficit Reduction Act, it became mandatory for some healthcare providers to comply, required education of staff regarding fraud and abuse laws, provided penalties for failure to comply, and provided incentives to state to adopt similar anti-fraud laws.

HIPAA provided more means for prosecution of fraud and abuse and increased penalties in addition to coordination of law enforcement at all levels and establishment of standardized practices. It provided greater means for enforcement, just as the Deficit Reduction Act did. HIPAA's goals include providing insurance portability, promote the use of medical savings account, decrease the costs of health care administration by simplifying insurance processes, and combating waste, fraud and abuse. HIPAA allows the government to mandate the use of standards for electronic exchange of health information and is known as Electronic Transactions and Code Sets Rule. Under HIPAA, a covered entity includes physicians, other healthcare providers, health plans, and healthcare clearinghouses who process claims. Business associates are those who do business with a covered entity. Both the covered entity and business associates must comply with HIPAA. There are two parts to HIPAA for security: the Privacy Rule and the Security Rule. The Privacy Rule refers to the concept of protected health information and its transmission and use. With the Privacy Rule only the minimal amount of patient information should be shared as required by law and no further information should be shared. The Security Rule refers to the concept of establishing protection for purposes of confidentiality and integrity of data.

Most investigations for fraud and abuse are initiated by complaints from current or former company employees who are then known as whistle-blowers. If a lawsuit develops from this it is known as qui tam action meaning that a private person stands in place of the government for the filing of charges. If the suit initiated by a whistle-blower is successfully prosecuted, that person will receive approximately 10% of the final award which could be considerable when awards are in the millions of dollars. Although there are laws that protect whistleblowers from retaliation, this is not always enforced.

Patient Protection and Affordable Care Act (PPACA) is the new healthcare reform legislation signed into law on March 30, 2010. It expands Medicaid eligibility, provides subsidies for insurance premiums for eligible persons and requires others to purchase their own health insurance if they have none, prohibits denial of healthcare coverage due to pre-existing conditions, and provides for intensified audits, investigations, penalties and limitations on payments to healthcare providers.

In 1996 the Health Care Financing Administration (HFCA), now known as the Center for Medicare and Medicaid Service (CMS) instituted the National **Correct Coding Initiative** (NNCCI) to assist in proper coding and billing of health care services, including issues regarding bundling. The CCI establishes rules for the determination of the correct methods to combine codes. CCI edits will inform the coder when combinations are not acceptable, such as the coding for an episiotomy when charging for vaginal delivery, which would be included in the cost of the vaginal delivery (global). Because of the National Correct Coding Initiative, you must be knowledgeable and be current in the field of coding and its applications through such things as study programs, seminars, research materials, and publications. CCI are published on a quarterly basis (Jan. 1–March 31; April 1–June 30; July 1–Sept. 30; Oct. 1–Dec. 31).

An additional piece of legislation is the Balanced Budget Act (BBA) of 1997 which requires the implementation of performance measures within the reimbursement/coding process. This type of legislation is important because of the effort to standardize the health record and the provision of health services through the development of performance measures and data sets. A performance measure inventory can be found at http://www.qualitymeasures.ahrq.gov/browse/browseorgsbyLtr.aspx?Letter=*Dozens.

Section 2.8: REGULATORY/GOVERNMENTAL AGENCIES

Many federal agencies are involved in the investigation and prosecution of fraud and abuse cases. Primary amongst these is the Office of Inspector General (OIG). In addition, the Department of Health and Human Services (HHS) is involved, as well as the Federal Bureau of Investigation (FBI), Department of Justice, Internal Revenue Service (IRS), Defense Criminal Investigative Services (DCIS), Drug Enforcement Agency (DEA), and the Post Office.

There are several additional agencies and programs which are used to audit and collect inappropriate and improper payments by governmental agencies to healthcare providers within OIG/CMS which are described below.

RECOVERY AUDIT CONTRACTORS (RACs): RACs are a recent creation of CMS which focus on recovery of improper payments based primarily on coding errors. RACs are entitled to 20% of the amount recovered. RACs were formed as part of Section 306 of the Medicare Prescription Drug, Improvement, and Modernization Act of 2003 (MMA) and was made permanent by Section 302 of the Tax Relief and Health Care Act of 2006 (TRHCA). In its initial 3-year trial, over $1 billion were collected due to improper payments by Medicare. There are two types of RAC reviews: the Automated (no medical record needed – just claims such as for double billing) and the Complex (medical record required). Reasons for recovery of funds by RACs included services that:

1. were found to be medically unnecessary
2. were incorrectly coded
3. had insufficient documentation in the record to support the treatment and services billed
4. contained other inconsistencies in the record and quality of care processes suggestive of billing that led to overpayment.

RACS will first send a demand letter containing some of the following: (1) Provider's identity, (2) Reason for the review, (3) List of claims, with findings, reasons for any denials, and amount of the overpayment for each claim, (4) Explanation of Medicare's right to charge interest on unpaid debts, (5) Instructions on paying the overpayments, (6) Explanation of the provider's right to submit a rebuttal statement and/or an appeal, (7) Description of the overpayment situation, including the reasons for the overpayment and suggested corrective actions, (8) Other demand letter requirements for written notifications, including the citation of the specific coverage, coding, or payment policies that the organization may have violated leading to the overpayment.

Following the initial demand letter, an appeal consists of the following: (1) Rebuttal, (2) redetermination, (3) reconsideration, (4) administrative law judge, (5) medicare appeal council, (6) US District Court.

Medicaid Integrity Program (MIPs) was created by the Deficit Reduction Act of 2005 to audit and collect Medicaid overpayments to healthcare providers with enforcement by Medicaid Integrity Contractors (MICs). Their role is to review provider actions, audit claims, identify overpayments; and educate providers, managed care entities, beneficiaries and others with respect to payment integrity and quality of care. The MIC mails a notification letter to the provider giving at least two weeks' notice before the audit is to begin.

Section 2.9: ELEMENTS OF A COMPLIANCE PROGRAM

A proper compliance program is the best insurance to proper reimbursement and office management practices. A proper compliance program should include
1. The development and institution of written standards for all aspects of the office management, including reimbursement and coding,
2. The selection of a compliance and security officer within the practice to develop and ensure institution and compliance with the written compliance program.
3. Provision of proper training to all staff and healthcare providers.
4. Established complaint process.
5. Enforcement policies for violations.
6. Audits and other evaluation techniques.
7. Investigation and remediation of violations and problems.

Section 2.10: OIG WORKPLAN

Each year, the Office of Inspector General publishes its work plan which highlights what coding areas will be focused on during that year for investigation. This is a valuable resource in that it can provide guidance as to proper coding so that proper measures and study can be taken by a healthcare provider to ensure that they are in compliance with those issues which may help thwart an audit or noncompliance (http://oig.hhs.gov/reports-and-publications/workplan/index.asp)

Section 2.11: AUDITING

Audits are reviews of practices and procedures to establish baselines and determine deviations, otherwise known as fraud, abuse, and/or omissions and mistakes. They can be initiated by external, internal, governmental or regulatory agencies with respect to possible fraud, abuse, or omissions/mistakes. The purpose of the auditing is to ensure proper compliance with rules and regulations with the ultimate purpose being the provision of quality healthcare. Auditing can involve coding as well as issues concerning reimbursement, privacy, legal, reimbursement, management, and compliance with regulatory requirements. Audits also ensure accuracy, consistency, timeliness and completeness.

Audits should be conducted on a regular basis which can be based on a certain percentage of charts reviewed or focused such as on certain specialties or doctors.   Audits can be either retrospective or prospective. A retrospective audit is done after a claim has been submitted; Prospective audits are done before the claim is submitted.

Audits should include auditing of the superbill on a regular basis to ensure that: (1) the codes are updated and current; (2) applicable and highly used codes are included on the superbill; (3) physicians and staff are selecting proper codes that are justified as medically necessary by the documentation in the patient's record.

Other reasons that may evoke the need to conduct an audit include rejected claims, OIG work plan, suspected problems due to staff comments, physician or administrative requests, and other changes in the reimbursement or coding processes.

REASONS FOR AUDITS: Reasons in the past for audits include:
1. Up-coding
2. Using a code that does not properly define the services provided.
3. Not documented not done services as reported.
4. Billing for services not performed.
5. Unnecessary treatment, not medically necessary which is not justified by diagnoses.
6. Too many codes of the same type
7. Performing disallowed procedures and billing them as allowed ones
8. Unbundling
9. Billing for procedures that are already covered under other global time periods.
10. Improper use of "multiple procedure codes."

PRE-AUDIT: Once the audit is approved and has full support of administration, requests must be made for the proper records and information. Charts and actual reports should be used for the audit. All staff, including physicians, should be notified to ensure their full cooperation.

It can be helpful to query staff and physicians about possible problem areas or issues to help guide the audit to determine if there are any particular areas of concern that should be focused on. This is particularly true of the billing and medical records department since employees may know of current issues that should be investigated. EOBs (explanation of benefits) can also be reviewed to investigate why claims were denied.

AUDIT: To conduct the audit full clinical records (either paper or electronic) need to be available. Forms can be developed to assist with collection of consistent and focused data from various people, including staff, physicians, and external agencies. The audit can be used to compare ICD-10 and CPT/HCPCS codes to ensure proper coding from the documentation, claim and EOBs completion and processing, determination of discrepancies, and to provide feedback to administration, staff and physicians through training, meetings and workshops.

POST AUDIT: The final report should contain the following:
1. Review of the purpose, objectives and methodology of the audit.
2. Report major coding deficiencies including coding errors and sources of errors.
3. The report containing the findings including areas of good practice, analysis of errors and recommendations.

DENIALS/APPEALS: Appeals are becoming a critical element in the reimbursement process since there are many external agencies which conduct audits and assess denials and penalties on healthcare providers. Because a healthcare provider may receive a notice of denial of payment or findings from an audit does not mean that they were not in compliance, so it is important that the staff/coder understand the process and are highly knowledgeable so that they can file proper appeals and ensure proper reimbursement and compliance for their healthcare providers.

CMS requires that RACs operate web-based systems so that providers who are involved in an audit will have secure online access to information that explains the status of their claims. CMS oversight will ensure that providers are not unduly burdened or second-guessed by the RACs. CMS will also require the RACs to identify and publish vulnerability analyses so that the provider community can better understand where mistakes are being made and have the opportunity to correct.

DOS AND DONTS FOR AUDITS:

1. Don't procrastinate by doing your response on the last day.
2. Don't expect to answer all of your audit complaints, but make an attempt to do each one.
3. Separate out each complaint into the "type of classification" usually by error type, diagnoses or procedure.
4. Don't throw away the demand letter or their audit report.
5. Less said the better. Responses should be written and carefully thought out.
6. Include documents that support your position.

CHAPTER 3
ICD-10 INTRODUCTION

You will learn the following objectives in this chapter:

Section 3.1: HISTORY OF ICD-10

ICD-10 was endorsed by the Forty-third World Health Assembly in May 1990 and was in application in 1994 throughout most of the world, except for United States although it is used for mortality purposes.

The first edition of ICD was known as the International List of Causes of Death originating in 1850. In 1948 WHO took over the responsibility for the ICD for the purposes of compilation of national mortality and morbidity statistics and subsequent classification of this data for the purposes of statistics, world-wide health management, research, records, storage of information, and compilation of national mortality and morbidity statistics throughout the world.

ICD has been regularly updated and changed to meet the greatly changing times within the healthcare field by WHO. Currently, the United States has been utilizing the 9th revision, while rest of the world has been using the ICD-10. One of the main reasons that United States has not adopted ICD-10 is because the revision needed to be altered for reimbursement and implementation purposes within United States, so the version ICD-10-CM needed to be developed.

The ICD is the largest classification system based on a hierarchial system. It classifies a wide variety of healthcare data with one of its main purposes being to provide statistics for healthcare research. In its purest form, ICD translates healthcare into numbers so that it can be processed in a meaningful way for reports and narratives.

Most importantly, the use of ICD codes was widely promoted by Medicare's requirement in the 1980's that they be used for all reporting and billing. Without the use of proper ICD codes, a healthcare provider would not be paid because the codes justify medical necessity of services provided.

Section 3.2: REASONS FOR CHANGE

With the ICD-10, countries are more able to track and respond to public health emergencies and utilize electronic records and SNOMED-CT more effectively. ICD-9 was no longer able to accomplish these goals because it lacked the ability to be more specific and detailed because it was running out of capacity and structure of numbers which, therefore, could not accommodate the vast advances and reimbursement issues in the healthcare field, specifically technology and quality, the continuous changes within diseases, and the ever-changing regulations and structure of healthcare practices, most specifically the electronic medical record. As a reflection of our times, ICD-10 is also better able to document and track terroristic attacks, biochemical attacks, and new and changing diseases through its alphanumeric format which allows for considerably more space for future revision without disruption of the numbering system.

ICD-10 provides greater compatibility and usability with SNOMED-CT. SNOMED-CT is the Systematized Nomenclature of Medicine -- Clinical Terms which is a computerized set of medical terminology covering diseases, findings, procedures, organisms, etc which, therefore, promotes the ability to electronically index, store, retrieve, and aggregate medical data from many healthcare sources which is contained within the electronic medical record (EMR) and is utilized with computer-assisted coding (CAC).

ICD-10 provides the ability of the United States to compare and share data about diseases with other countries who are utilizing ICD-10 now which promotes better public health surveillance and research. It also provides better measures of patient care quality since it is more attune to new technologies and procedures since it adds more detail and expands codes for medical complications and safety issues, particularly for the top causes of mortality and diseases, even those related to terroristic attacks. This also promotes greater response to reimbursement issues, such as medical necessity, and less errors; therefore, promoting better management and institutional performance.

ICD-10 provides the ability to rate the severity of diseases which is critically important in the outcomes of the patient's care and assessment of institutional and practice practices.

External cause of injury codes detailing external factors that produced the injury are also much more detailed in ICD-10-CM which help in ensuring injury prevention and developing safety programs, including in the workplace and for violent crimes.

ICD-10-CM index, tabular, guidelines, and general equivalence mapping files on the National Center for Health Statistics Web site at: www.cdc.gov/nchs/about/otheract/icd9/icd10cm.htm.

General Equivalence Mappings (GEMs) are provided from various sources which help with crosswalking from ICD-9 codes to ICD-10 codes although it must be strongly noted that, like with any type of translation, the codes are not equivalent as there are many differences and additions/deletions which compromise the accuracy of crosswalking.

Section 3.3: ICD-10 DESCRIPTION

ICD-10-CM is an acronym which stands for "International Classification of Diseases, 9th Revision, Clinical Modification." ICD-10-CM is a clinical modification (CM) of the World Health Organization's ICD-10 for use within the United States in the same fashion as the ICD-9-CM and is maintained by the U.S. National Center for Health Statistics. ICD-10-PCS is developed by the Center for Medicare and Medicaid Services (CMS) and is used by hospitals to code for procedures and services that are performed as inpatient. CMS also provides regular updates and information which can be found through the Correct Coding Initiative and Federal Register, as well as many other sources such as insurance companies, state health departments, and organizations.

With ICD-10-CM, there are two sections, ICD-10 and ICD-10-PCS. ICD-10 is reminiscent of the traditional Volumes 1 and 2 from ICD-9 and ICD-10-PCS is reminiscent of Volume 3 which provided codes for in-hospital procedures. ICD-10-PCS codes are alphanumeric codes comprised of 7 characters.

There are more than 68,000 codes in the ICD-10-CM compared to the approximately 13,000 ICD-9-CM diagnosis codes. There are more than 87,000 procedure codes in the ICD-10-PCS. Both of these numbers demonstrate that clearly there is greater specificity in the ICD-10-CM and PCS.

The structure of the ICD-10 is similar to ICD-9 in that there are three volumes with chapters and categories. There are 21 chapters in ICD-10 whereas there were only 17 in ICD-9. There are two new chapters, Chapter VII "Diseases of the eyelid and adnexa" and Chapter VIII "Diseases of the ear and mastoid process". Other chapters have new and expanded names. Some chapters, such as "symptoms, signs and ill-defined conditions" have increased by more than 300%.

The ICD-10-CM book is divided into three volumes:
> Volume 1: Tabular List of Diseases and Injuries
> Volume 2: Alphabetic Index to Diseases
> Volume 3: Tabular List of and Alphabetic Index to Procedures

These will be described later in this module and throughout all of the modules.

First, although there are three volumes in ICD-10-CM books, for physician coding only the first two volumes are used. The third volume is for coding of procedures in the hospital. Many ICD-10-CM books do not contain a third volume because this is used strictly for inpatient hospital coding and is not used for physician coding. Therefore, there is no reason for a person to pay additional monies for a book with three volumes if they are not going to be coding for inpatient hospital procedures. For this course which focuses on coding for the physician offices, we are only interested in the first two volumes. It is advised that you do not study for the inpatient hospital coding unless you are going to be doing inpatient hospital coding because it does differ from physician coding. Studying for inpatient hospital coding can be confusing when preparing to take the test for physician coding and may result in lost points and possible test failure.

Section 3.4: DIFFERENCES BETWEEN ICD-10-CM BOOKS

There are many versions of the ICD-10-CM book published by various companies with many differences. It is recommended when you take the national coding exams that you use a regular book and not any described as expert or otherwise. In fact, alternative versions may not be allowed on exams so do not jeopardize your chances of passing your national exam by using an alternative book. The reason for this is that some of those differences could affect the outcome of your test because you may not have access to some important information. During this course, you will learn about what are the most helpful and important attributes to look for in an ICD-10-CM book.

Also, there are different publishers and different features to each type of book. One of these differences is that some publishers will put the alphabetic index first and the tabular index second. Note, at the beginning of this section, however, that Volume 1 is known as the Tabular List and Volume 2 is known as the Alphabetic Index. Even though these volumes may be switched in the order of their presentation, it still remains that Volume 1 is the Tabular List and Volume 2 is the Alphabetic Index. It is important to emphasize that, because of this, you should become familiar with the use of your book, particularly before testing, so that you can easily and quickly find your way through the book without confusion as it could result in errors and lost time which are not desirable during a national test.

Section 6.5: DIFFERENCES BETWEEN ICD-9 AND ICD-10 BOOKS

Although the differences between the ICD-9 and ICD-10 codes will be discussed and illustrated throughout this entire book, a general presentation is provided now.

- There are 21 chapters in ICD-10 but in ICD-9 there were only 17.
- ICD-10 codes are alphanumeric rather than the ICD-9 where most codes were only numeric.
- There are additional characters possible for codes in ICD-10, up to seven, whereas the most characters possible in ICD-9 were five.
- Codes in ICD-10 now specify laterality which was not available ICD-9 codes.
- There is the use of a placeholder denoted by X which is used when a space is not filled in with other characters but rather the X is used to hold the place for future use when additional expansion may be needed for codes.
- There are full code descriptions in ICD-10 rather than the breakdown of common fourth and fifth characters into one box which were then applied to numerous codes as seen in ICD-9.
- There are now combination codes for poisonings and their causes in ICD-10 rather than the additional E codes for causes that were used in ICD-9.
- There is greater specification within codes such as pregnancy codes further distinguished by trimesters for ICD-10.
- V and E codes of the ICD-9 are now incorporated into the main code classification in ICD-10.
- ICD-10 does classify some codes by anatomic site such as injuries which are first coded by site and then by injury; ICD-9 classified by injury.

- There are new separate chapters in ICD-10 for eye and ear conditions which did not exist in ICD-9.
- Changes in time frames in ICD-10 for some codes such as MI which are now 4 weeks instead of 8 weeks.
- There are many reclassifications of diseases and conditions to other chapters in ICD-10 which differ from where the codes were placed in ICD-9 including more use of combination codes.
- Postoperative complications are now included in each chapter by procedure-body system in ICD-10 rather than in their own section at the end of Volume 1 as they were in ICD-9.
- In ICD-10 there are now two types of exclude notes. Exclude 1 indicates "not coded here" in which the excluded code cannot be listed with the condition described in the original code. Exclude 2 indicates "not included here" as it is not part of the condition described in the code.

Section 3.6: DESCRIPTION OF VOLUMES

ICD-10-CM has an alphabetical index and tabular list similar to those of ICD-9-CM including indentations and use of sections, categories, and subcategories which creates the familiar hierarchical system. The main terms are in bold.

There are two parts to the ICD-10-CM alphabetical index which are the index to diseases and injury and index to external causes of injury. As with the ICD-9 the table of drugs and chemicals and the neoplasm table are contained with the alphabetical index. There no longer is a table for hypertension.

Volume 1 is known as the Tabular List of Diseases and Injuries. This is where the codes are located. Again, it does not matter where the book organizes the volumes, Volume 1 remains as the Tabular List and lists the actual codes. The Alphabetic Index is Volume 2 and contains alphabetical listing of conditions as well as the Neoplasm Table and, Index for External Causes of Injury, and Table of Drugs and Chemicals.

HIERARCHIAL SYSTEM: The Tabular List is organized in a hierarchical classification system. Understanding and properly using the hierarchical system is critical to proper coding, so be sure to understand this system of indentations, highlighting, and other notations that will be discussed as the means to classifying diseases and injuries.

The hierarchical systems are categorized by alphanumeric characters. Codes can vary from three to seven characters. The various characters can symbolize details of diseases, injuries, and conditions which prompt the need for medical care. These will be discussed within each section where it is applicable.

RULE: A critical rule involving the use of the hierarchical system in ICD-10-CM coding is **CODE TO THE HIGHEST LEVEL OF SPECIFICITY,** which will be discussed below.

Section 3.7: CLASSIFICATIONS

The hierarchical system is based on classifications (or subdivisions). Again, it is not as important to remember the exact definition of what each level signify but rather to understand the application. The change to a different level of classification is indicated by indentations within the Tabular List.

The first subdivision is by **CHAPTER.**

Volume 1 consists of 21 chapters, rather than the 17 of ICD-9. Chapters are based on body system or condition. The first character is alphabetical but the remaining characters may be either alphabetical or numeric.

These chapters are:

1.	Infectious and Parasitic Diseases	A00-B99
2.	Neoplasms	C00-D49
3.	Diseases of the Blood and Blood-Forming Organs	D50-D89
4.	Endocrine, Nutritional, and Metabolic Diseases, and Immunity Disorders	E00-E89
5.	Mental & Behavioral Disorders	F01-F99
6.	Diseases of the Nervous System And Sense Organs	G00-G99
7.	Disease of Eye & Adnexa	H00-H59
8.	Diseases of Ear & Mastoid Process	H60-H59
9.	Diseases of the Circulatory System	I00-I99
10.	Diseases of the Respiratory System	J00-J99
11.	Diseases of the Digestive System	K00-K95
12.	Diseases of the Skin and Subcutaneous Tissue	L00-L99
13.	Diseases of the Musculoskeletal System & Connective Tissue	M00-M99
14.	Diseases of the Genitourinary System	N00-N99
15.	Complications of the Pregnancy, Childbirth, and Puerperium	O00-O9A
16.	Certain Conditions Originating in the Perinatal Period	P00-P96
17.	Congenital Malformations, Deformations & Chromosomal Abnormalities	Q00-Q99
18.	Symptoms, Signs, and Abnormal Clinical & Laboratory Findings, Not elsewhere classified	R00-R99
19.	Injury, Poisoning & Certain Other Consequences of External Causes	S00-T88
20.	External Causes of Morbidity	V01-Y99
21.	Factors Influencing Health Status & Contact With Health Services	Z00-Z99

Codes are further broken down by categories, subcategories and valid codes. SUBCATEGORIES are indicated by either four or five characters. It is important to remember to code to **THE HIGHEST LEVEL OF SPECIFICITY RULE** by putting the correct number of characters required for a code. There are notes and indications at the bottom of each page to denote when an additional character is required.

X is used as a placeholder in some codes which allows for future expansion of codes.

Section 3.8: CHARACTERS

ICD-10 has a new name, "International Statistical Classification of Diseases and Related Health Problems".

The first most important concept is that almost all of the codes were only numeric in ICD-9-CM but are alphanumeric in ICD-10-CM and structured on a hierarchical system. It is very important that the correct number of characters are applied or payment will be denied and the coding will be wrong.

The importance of learning this hierarchical system can be seen in the selection of a wrong code by not following the hierarchical system which results in serious errors which will be seen repeatedly throughout the modules as we go more in depth. In other words, if the condition requires the use of four characters as directed by the ICD-10-CM book, then four characters must be coded. The same for five characters and so forth for all characters.

DETERMING CHARACTER NOTATIONS: The first character for ICD-10 codes is always alphabetical. All letters of the alphabet are used with the exception of U which has been reserved by WHO for assignment of new diseases of uncertain etiology and for drug-resistant bacteria.

The remaining characters can be either alphabetical or numeric with the exception of the second character which is always numeric. Seventh characters are used to denote encounters or sequelae for injuries and external causes.

As with ICD-9, the period is placed after the first three characters.

Do not neglect to include the proper number of characters when coding because it is wrong as previously noted. For example, do not use only four characters when five characters are required.

First, there are notations in the tabular list which indicate the proper number of characters, as well as sometime an indication of which specific character should be used, which will be discussed further in later chapters. These notations can include a notation by the side of various codes that indicate the need for a fourth or fifth character.

Second, most additional characters are indicated with full descriptions following the initial code. For example, Multiple myeloma (C90.0) has further specification such as C90.00 for multiple myeloma not having achieved remission, C90.01 in remission and C90.02 in relapse.

Third, in the alphabetical index, a hyphen (-) is listed after some codes to indicate that additional characters are required.

> **IMPORTANT! When it is noted that a character needs to be added, be sure to add the character in its proper place.**

In other words, a notation will indicate if a fourth or fifth character needs to be listed so be sure that your code has the proper number of characters. The first character is the third character to the left of the period. The second character is the second character to the left of the period. The third character is the first character to the left of the period. The fourth character is the first character to the right of the period. The fifth character is the second character to the right of the period and so on. If a character is required in a specific location, but there are there no values associated with a previous character space assigned yet, then "x" is used as a placeholder. For example, T38.4X1. The X does not represent any value yet but a seventh character is required so the "X" holds the space to ensure proper use of character spacing.

BE CAREFUL! Do not transpose characters. Again, using the example above, do not enter T37.4X5 when the code is T37.5X4. It in these transpositions that many coding errors are made.

An additional source of common errors in coding is selecting the code from the wrong line. This is a significant problem and be sure you are overly cautious concerning this selection from the wrong line as it is extremely easy to do. This error occurs due to the complex and extensive hierarchical system of coding as previously explained and will be discussed further in discussion about the alphabetical index. In other words, be sure that you did not go into another section of classification and indentation. This is particularly a problem when you change to another column or page. The alphabetical index for ICD-10 has tried to eliminate this problem by adding grey bars along the side of the pages which indicate when categories begin and when another code is listed under that code or has its own subcategory.

Section 3.9: DESCRIPTION OF VOLUME 2

Volume 2 is known as the Alphabetical Index. Again, this may be listed second in the ICD-10-CM book which is why it is known as Volume 2; however, some books are printed with the Volume 2 listed first.

Volume 2 is divided into:
1. Alphabetical Index listing diseases and injuries.
2. Table of Drugs and Chemicals.
3. Alphabetic Index to External Causes of Injury and Poisoning (E codes).

There are some basic critical rules to remember about utilizing Volume 2.

RULE: NEVER CODE DIRECTLY FROM VOLUME 2!

If there are discrepancies or debate regarding selection of the proper code, the ICD-10-CM book is used as the final authority, the basis for all coding decisions, and the tabular index is the final authority. The ICD-10-CM book is very clear and precise. Therefore, if either the Tabular List or the Alphabetical Index provides direction on selecting the proper code, then you must follow these directions. When coding, always remember – YOU MUST USE THE ICD-10-CM CODING BOOK TO JUSTIFY YOUR SELECTIONS, so if someone came two years later questioning why you selected certain codes, then you would need to demonstrate a rationale from the ICD-10-CM code book for why you chose the code you did.

It is important to remember this because oftentimes the Alphabetical Index will provide instructions on selecting on the proper code. If the Index tells you to do so, then do so. Do not interpret (misinterpret) the codes because of information you may think you know that contradicts the information in the ICD-10-CM book. If you have a disagreement with codes as they are, the proper place to ask those question is not when you are coding to bill, but by addressing the questions to CMS.

Section 3.10: SELECTION OF CODES FROM VOLUME 2

MAIN TERMS: Of course, the alphabetical index is set up alphabetically; however, there are some idiosyncrasies that can complicate finding the correct code. Basically, the index is set up in a hierarchical system beginning with main terms which can be based on anatomical site, diseases, eponyms, conditions, general nouns and adjectives. These terms are bolded. An eponym is a term named after a person which is common in the medical field, such as Parkinson's disease and Lou Gehrig's Disease. The main terms are also listed at the top of each page, much as it would be found in a dictionary. It is important to acknowledge general terms because many codes are listed here and not elsewhere. Examples of general terms include "failure", "disease", "examination", "disturbance", "disorder", "dependence, "problem", etc.

IMPORTANT!   In the alphabetical index for ICD-10-CM, if there is a hyphen (-) listed at the end of a code entry, this indicates that additional characters are needed.

SUBTERMS: Below the main terms there is usually a listing of subterms which are further elaborations (modifications) of the main term. Under subterms, you will find more subterms (carryovers) which are further elaborations (modifications) of the subterms, which forms the hierarchical system of the ICD-10-CM codes. To create the hierarchical system, these subterms are indented under the term that it is connected to. For example, if you locate contusion in the alphabetical index, you will see there are many subterms, but that the indentation of the terms varies. The subterms, "with", "abdomen", "adnexa", are the first set of subterms and are indented but are the farthest indentation to the left under the main term, "contusion." Notice under "with" that there subterms which are further indented, which include "crush injury", "dislocation", etc. This means that these terms are all a subterm of "contusion". Now notice that under "contusion, with, internal injury", there are more subterms which are further indented, such as "heart", "kidney," and "liver". These are subterms of "contusion", but only of "contusion, with, internal injury". They are not subterms of "abdomen" or "adnexa" under "contusion".

Due to this hierarchical system, you will find that the terms are categorized in several ways. First, the subterms are categorized alphabetically. Most of the subterms can be found this way. But this becomes complicated because there are subterms under subterms which disrupts the alphabetical nature of this index.

Second, subterms under other subterms will be listed alphabetically, but this disrupts the original alphabetical indexing for the first subterm. In other words, you will have multiple alphabetical indices, so there are alphabetical indices contained within other alphabetical indices which, again, form the hierarchical nature of ICD-10-CM coding. Let's examine our example again of "contusion." Locate "arm" under "contusion". You will find that it has a couple of subterms further indented under it. This means that "lower" and "upper" are referring to a contusion on the arm and not any other term, such as abdomen or adnexa. This process of indentations is very important to understand and to use properly; otherwise, you may be selecting your codes from the wrong terms.

Third, as noted above, there are other subterms that disrupt the alphabetical indexing. These oftentimes are connecting terms or nouns other than diseases, conditions, or anatomic sites. There are a variety of these terms that occur commonly throughout the alphabetical index and they do disrupt the alphabetical listing but they are oftentimes very important in helping to find the correct code. In fact, if you cannot find your term alphabetically, you may find it under one of these terms. These general terms that are used throughout the alphabetical index include "with", "due to", "during", "following", "involving", "in", "secondary to", "with mention of", "complicated by", "management affected by", "administration of", "adjustment," etc. Therefore, you must be check in several places for a term: (1) traditional alphabetical ordering, (2) subterms under terms, (3) and general terms.

Therefore, when a term is indented under another term, it means that it is a subdivision or modifier of the term under which it is indented. This can vary from a few subterms to a lot. This is where the use of the alphabetical index becomes tricky, mainly because there are so many subterms and indentations that it becomes difficult to know if you are under the right term. For this reason, it becomes important that you take time to search through the main terms and subterms to be sure that you have found the right code and did not miss it somewhere.

Therefore, when you are looking for a code in the alphabetical index, you may have to look in several places and you must be sure that you do not get into the wrong main term or subterms. To achieve this, you must keep track of indentations and the alphabetical indexing, so if you are looking under terms that go from A to C to F, etc., and then you notice that the next term is B, then you know that you are no longer under the term you were originally looking under. For example, if you are looking for "pregnancy, complicated by", and you are then looking under "hemorrhage, threatened abortion" but you notice that you are looking at "h's" again, under hepatitis and hypertension, then you know that you have gone out of the subterms you wanted because "h" does not come before "t" in the alphabet.

Section 3.11: Z CODES

Z codes are what used to be Y codes. They are a supplementary classification system located at the end of the Tabular List in Volume. They are a listing of "Factors Influencing Health Status and Contact with Health Services." They contain a large variety of codes which are applied to services which do not meet the typical description of diseases and conditions as listed in the Tabular Index itself. These codes can be found in the Alphabetical Index for the tabular codes. These will be discussed later in their own packet. Oftentimes in ICD-10-CM codes the factors influencing health status and contact are included in the core code rather than having a separate code.

Section 3.12: S, T, V AND Y CODES

S, T, V, and Y codes are what used to be E codes. They are a supplementary classification system that is now before the Z codes in Volume 1. They are the supplementary classification of External Causes of Injury and Poisoning. Oftentimes in ICD-10-CM codes the external causes of injury and poisoning are included in the core code rather than having a separate code.

CHAPTER 4
ICD-10 CODING CONVENTIONS

You will learn the following objectives in this chapter:

A. Guidelines
    1. Placeholder
    2. Combination Codes
    3. Laterality
    4. New Codes
B. Late Effects
C. Medical Care Complications
    1. Postsurgical Complications
    2. Prosthetics/Grafts
    3. Infections
    4. Transplants
    5. Other
D. Code First
E. Cross-Referencing
F. Inclusion Notes/Nonessential Modifiers
G. Exclusion notes
H. Punctuation
    1. Parentheses
    2. Colon
    3. Square Brackets
    4. Slanted Brackets
I. Abbreviations
    1. NEC
    2. NOS

Section 4.1: GUIDELINES

PLACEHOLDERS: New to ICD-10-CM is the use of placeholders. X is always used as the placeholder in that it holds the place of that position for future use so that the structure of the code is not distorted, because if a character is required in the seventh position then it must be in the seventh position and not moved to fifth or sixth just because there are no values yet for those positions.

COMBINATION CODES: There are now more combination codes in the ICD-10 in which the cause and condition are coded together.

Combination Codes for Conditions and Common Symptoms:

- I25.110, Arteriosclerotic heart disease of native coronary artery with unstable angina pectoris

- K50.013, Crohn's disease of small intestine with fistula
- K71.51, Toxic liver disease with chronic active hepatitis with ascites

Combination Codes for Poisonings and the External Cause

- T39.011, Poisoning by aspirin, accidental (unintentional)
- T39.012, Poisoning by aspirin, intentional self harm
- T39.013, Poisoning by aspirin, assault
- T39.014, Poisoning by aspirin, undetermined

LATERALITY: ICD-10 codes are now more specific about the area of the body involved including right or left, such as left lower eyelid.

- C50.212, Malignant neoplasm of upper-inner quadrant of left female breast
- H02.835, Dermatochalasis of left lower eyelid
- I80.01, Phlebitis and thrombophlebitis of superficial vessels of right lower extremity
- L89.213, Pressure ulcer of right hip, stage III

NEW CODES: There are many new codes for conditions that did not have a specific code in ICD-9, e.g., Chronic fatigue syndrome (G93.3), chronic intractable pain (R52.1) and stress NOS (Z73.3.).

In addition to new codes, some codes have been moved to other chapters, e.g., transient cerebral ischemic attacks and related syndromes are now in the chapter for "Diseases of the Nervous System," rather than the circulatory chapter of the ICD-9.

Section 4.2: LATE EFFECTS: Late effects are now coded in the chapter to which they apply anatomically e,g, sequelae of injury of nerve of lower limb (T93.4). A late effect is a residual or sequelae that has continued after the treatment for the causal or etiological condition has concluded. Residuals and sequelae are conditions caused by another condition (etiology).

Late effects may be temporary or permanent. There is no time limit to determine a late effect; it will depend upon the condition and the patient.

Late effects in the alphabetical index of the ICD-10 book instruct to look under "sequelae". You can also find late effects listed under specific conditions, e.g., under hemiplegia there is a listing for "late effects or residual".

Section 4.3: MEDICAL CARE COMPLICATIONS

POSTSURGICAL COMPLICATIONS: Many postsurgical complications are now coded at the end of the chapter to which they are associated anatomically instead of in the last chapter of the coding book, e.g., vomiting following gastrointestinal surgery (K91.0) or infection due to foreign object left during a procedure (T81.6). However, some non-specific disorders are still coded in the last chapter, such as shock and air embolism.

Medical care complications are conditions and complications that result from medical care and are known as misadventures. Codes for complications of medical care are only used for unanticipated/undesirable conditions that result from the medical care itself; not for common and anticipated conditions of medical care. In other words, swelling is a common aftercare condition of a surgery, so it would not be coded as a complication of medical care. On the other hand, if a patient has an indwelling catheter and develops an infection, this would be considered a complication of the medical care and would be coded because, although infections do occur, it is not an acceptable outcome of medical care.   There is no time limit on when conditions and complications of medical care can develop.

Medical care complications can be found in the alphabetical index under a variety of terms, including the complication itself, postsurgical, complications, medical care, and surgical procedures.

PROSTHETICS/GRAFTS: A common category that can produce postsurgical complications involve prosthetics and grafts. Prosthetics include a wide variety of devices and implants, such as heart valves, pacemaker, catheters, shunts, electrodes, contraceptive device, colostomy, screws, nails, and plates, . Medical care complications can include breakdown, displacement, perforation, protrusion, leakage, or obstruction by the devices. Although these conditions do occur, it is not an acceptable outcome of the surgery. These are coded as complications, prosthesis and under the specific prosthesis such as graft. Usually T codes are used to code for these.

INFECTION: Although infections also do occur from medical care, again they are not acceptable outcomes. They can be coded with T codes also such as T81.4.

TRANSPLANTS: Transplants oftentimes result in medical care complications and are coded by anatomic site; however, complications are only coded if they impair the functioning of the transplant. T86 codes are used to code for these complications.

OTHER: Other medical care complication codes include postoperative shock, hemorrhage, puncture or laceration, disruption of wound, foreign body left in the operation site, emphysema, non-healing surgical wound, air embolism, and infusion reactions.

Section 4.4: CODE FIRST/USE ADDITIONAL CODE

There is the use of "code also" and "use additional code if desired" in ICD-10 as there was in ICD-9. The use of the terms "due to" and "resulting in" do indicate causal relationship, but the use of terms "with", "with mention of", "associated with", and "in" do not necessarily indicate a causal relationship. The use of term "and" means they are not connected.

Section 4.5: CROSS REFERENCES

Under main terms and subterms, there are many cross-references in the alphabetical index which are extremely helpful. Cross references may be denoted by the terms, "see also," "see condition," etc. followed by the term of where to check or there may be a reference or duplication of terms. For example:

1. You can find references to pregnancy conditions under pregnancy, labor and delivery, postpartum, antepartum, etc.
2. You can find references to a condition under its own name, anatomical site, modifier, or condition, such as cortical blindness which can be found under cortical or blindness. If you look in the alphabetical index under cortical, you will see a note that says "see also condition." This means to check under "blindness."

When the alphabetical index makes a cross-reference, be sure to use the exact term. For instance, when a cross reference says, "see condition," it does not mean to look up the word "condition," but to look for the condition, such as "failure" for heart failure.

When the index makes references or notations, you must follow the directions completely. Do not alter or re-interpret what the alphabetical index or even the tabular list tells you to do. Follow it precisely. This point will be emphasized repeatedly throughout the packets.

Section 4.6: INCLUSION NOTES/NONESSENTIAL MODIFIERS

You will also find terms in the alphabetical index in parenthesis. These are known as nonessential modifiers because they do not need to be described in the patient's chart to allow for the use of this code. They are simply providing extra information to assist in more accurate coding.

Inclusion notes are similar to nonessential modifiers in that they do not exclude the use of codes to conditions not listed, but rather are simply providing more information. In other words, if a condition is not listed in the include notes of a code, the code may still be the correct code. The inclusions notes simply provide additional information to assist in the selection of the proper code, but again, do not preclude the use of the code for a condition that is not listed in the inclusion notes.

Again, if you have determined that this is the correct code from the use of the diagnostic statements provided by the physician and the use of the alphabetical index and tabular index but it is not described in these terms, you will still use these codes. Remember, inclusion notes do not exclude the use of the code for other descriptive diagnostic statements.

Section 4.7: EXCLUSIONS NOTES

There are two new exclude notes definitions.

Excludes 1 note means "not coded here" which means the excluded code is never used with the original code, they are exclusive of each other, i.e. they cannot exist together at the same time.

Excludes 2 note means "not included here" which means the excluded condition is not coded as part of the original code; therefore, if the patient does have both conditions they can both be coded but they are not coded as part of each other.

Exclusion notes are critical! They must be read in detail and followed precisely. The term

EXCLUDE is bolded in the ICD-10-CM book. Again, details are critical in coding and this is one detail that is! The exclusion note will apply to all codes within that main code.

Section 4.8: PUNCTUATION

PARENTHESIS: As discussed earlier, there are nonessential modifiers (supplementary words) which are additional information provided by the ICD-10-CM book to assist in proper coding which are included in parenthesis. Remember those that these do not exclude the use of this code for other diagnostic descriptions that are not included in the parenthesis.

COLON: A colon indicates additional modifiers of a term and these modifiers are indented below the term they modify.

SQUARE BRACKETS: Square brackets in the tabular list enclose alternate wording for a diagnostic description, including synonyms, abbreviations and phrases. In the alphabetical index, brackets are used to identify manifestation codes such as nephrosis in amyloidosis E85.4 [N08].

Section 4.9: ABBREVIATIONS

NEC: Not elsewhere classified. This category of codes is used when other information is provided about a code, but there is no specific code for it. This is usually indicated by the use of an "8" in the fourth position. It is also known as "other specified". For example, notice in code E22.8, it states "other". Again, this indicates that the specific site was not listed by itself and so this code contains a number of groups or sites. While this is the common practice of using 8 to signify "other", it does not mean that the description of the codes always follow this protocol, so always be sure to read the descriptions carefully. "8" can be used for other factors such as anatomic site.

NOS: Not otherwise specified. This category of codes is used when no other information is available and is usually indicated by the use of a "9". Notice also that the code's description may also say "unspecified", which means the same thing in referring to there being no further information provided. For example, see code D27.9 or D26.9 where the term "unspecified" is used. While this is the common practice, it does not mean that the description of the codes always follow this protocol of assigning "9" to NOS, so always be sure to read the descriptions carefully. "9" can be used for other factors such as anatomic site. Sometimes the NOS description is used in the beginning of a subcategory but only because the entire category is the last category.

CHAPTER 5
ICD-10 BASIC CODING GUIDELINES

You will learn the following in this chapter:

A. Basic coding guidelines and rules
     1. Medical Necessity
     2. Not documented, not done
B. Proper Coding with ICD-10
C. Multiple Codes
     1. Etiology/Manifestation
     2. Additional Codec/Code Also
     3. Code First
D. Combination Codes
E. Sequencing
F. Comorbidities and complications
G. Symptoms
H. Rule outs

Section 5.1: BASIC CODING GUIDELINES AND RULES

MEDICAL NECESSITY: The ICD-10-CM codes are used to prove medical necessity….this is a critical term on which all payment is based which is why providing the proper ICD-10-CM code is important. Services provided will not be paid if the ICD-10-CM code does not prove that the service was necessary. For example, if a patient is seen for a fractured leg and receives a stress test for a heart problem, then this service will be denied because it was not related to the care of the fracture. This is a huge problem nowadays as there are practices that will charge for services, such as tests, which they either do not provide or which should not have been provided because the patient's condition did not require it.

NOT DOCUMENTED, NOT DONE: This means that you can only code what the physician or healthcare provider has stated in the reports and notes within the patient's file. You cannot re-interpret, change, or ignore what is written in the patient's record.   So, you cannot code more than or less than what the physician or healthcare provider has written.

If you find when you are attempting to code a report you cannot make a coding choice because the information is not clear, you can make queries of the physician at that time for the purpose of clarification. For example, if a report states that a patient is on insulin but the physician does not classify it as Type I, you may want to inquire of the physician if the patient is Type I diabetic.

Remember – **NOT DOCUMENTED, NOT DONE.** You can only code what the physician has reported and you cannot make your own interpretations. If a physician tells you he meant to put certain information in the report but failed to do so, then explain to him that in the future he must be sure to include it but you cannot code it unless it was in the signed final report.

When you are coding for a physician, you should derive your codes from the physician's statements as he determines the diagnosis, not you. This is a part of the "not documented, not done" concept because the physician must provide the information and make the diagnosis.

So, **NEVER** give a patient a diagnosis they do not have, and you can ensure that by never coding a diagnosis unless the physician has stated it which is a basic rule of coding, **NOT DOCUMENTED, NOT DONE.** This is one area of coding that causes enormous problems for nurses as they are accustomed to always trying to figure out what is wrong with the patient, but coders cannot do that – two completely different scenarios. So, nurses in particular, but others as well, may try to determine diagnosis, but remember that only the physician can do this, so avoid the urge (despite any available information or verbal directives) to select a code based on your making a diagnosis and not the physician's written statements.

This also applies to the physician making a report, signing a report, and then the physician wishing to later verbally add to the report after the bill has been sent so that a higher code can be billed. If the physician did not put the information in the report, it cannot be billed. This is poor practice and is a red flag for auditors and government agencies.

What can be done for situations where physicians are not reporting proper information to ensure correct billing and coding is that the coder should be involved in the education and training of the physician (and all office and healthcare staff) with regards to report formats and what they need to include in their reports to receive proper reimbursement. This education and training will then ensure that the proper procedures will be followed in the future and prevent future failures to receive full reimbursement.

Section 5.2: PROPER CODING WITH ICD-10-CM

There are many ways that the ICD-10-CM book provides valuable information in the selection of the codes. For this reason, you must follow the book's direction closely. Do not re-interpret what it tells you to do, nor disregard any information it provides.

How informative the ICD-10-CM book is will depend on the book you are using. Some books provide not only inclusion and exclusion notes, but also coding guideline notes, definitions, and references. Some provide additional table formatting. It is for this reason you should become familiar with the structure of your coding books before the national exam to ensure that you can quickly and easily find the correct codes and utilize all of the advantages that a book may offer.

IMPORTANT! At the front of the book are coding guidelines which are very helpful in further explaining the proper use of codes and are very helpful, especially during testing.

The process of selecting the right code begins with locating it in the alphabetical index. However, remember that you never select a code from the alphabetical index. This is because there are many notes, as are being described in this packet and others, which are listed in the tabular list and which are critical to the selection of the correct code.

Therefore, begin by searching for what you believe is the main term from the diagnostic statement (located on superbills or ideally in charts or reports). If you cannot find your code under this term, then pick the next best term to describe the condition. If that does not work, continue through the terms you have until you find the correct code. If you still cannot find the correct code, then you should think of terms that are similar to the terms describing the patient's condition.

Remember in our description of the structure of the book and conventions that you need to look for other terms as well, such as "with", "due to", "disease," etc. You may also need to follow instructions within the ICD-10-CM book, such as "see" and "see also."

Remember, follow the instructions within the alphabetical index and tabular list precisely. Correct coding depends heavily on the following of details precisely from the ICD-10-CM book.

If codes are listed in the alphabetical index in parenthesis, do not use them as the selected code. These signify other information about the code which varies by the codes, but is never the actual code to be selected.

Section 5.3: MULTIPLE CODES

Several diagnostic statements may be present in a report and linked to each other (such as etiology and manifestation) as per the physician's statement, so they will either be coded together as one code or as multiple codes. You can find referrals to code additional diagnostic statements with another code in either the Tabular List or Alphabetical Index.

Multiple coding means that more than one code is required to code for a condition:

(1) ETIOLOGY/MANIFESTATION: There may be an etiology code and a manifestation code which would both need to be coded. Etiology is the cause and manifestation is the condition that results from the etiology. Usually the etiology will be listed first in reporting the codes and the manifestation second.

(2) ADDITIONAL CODE/CODE ALSO: There may be a notation in the ICD-10-CM book that states "use additional code, if desired" or "code also." Ignore the "desired" term; you must code the additional code. You must be careful to ensure that you find any of these notations, even if you have to search back to the beginning of the section because the additional code must be coded, if known. For example, J13 instructs to code also associated lung abscess. Most use additional code listings include a category now for tobacco use (Z72.0) such as J37, Chronic laryngitis.

(3) CODE FIRST: Another notation in the ICD-10-CM book is "code first underlying disease." You must be careful to ensure that you find any of these notations, even if you have to search back to the beginning of the section because the additional code must be coded, if known. This notation is particularly important in that it is providing you information about the order of the codes. For example, J12 instructs to code first associated influenza.

On occasion with multiple coding, information may not be provided in the report which allows for coding the second code. Under these circumstances, you cannot code the extra code. If the second code cannot be coded, however, this may result in denial of payment since the medical necessity of the services provided may not be justified, so it is important that physicians provide all the necessary information so that the correct code can be selected.

Section 5.4: COMBINATION CODES

Combination codes are comprised of one code that contains more than one diagnostic statement and does not require coding of any additional codes.

In contrast to ICD-9, in ICD-10-CM there are more combination codes which then do not require the coding of additional codes, such as diabetes codes, e.g. E10.21 for type diabetes mellitus with diabetic nephropathy. This also applies to poisonings, such as T41.291 for accidental poisoning by general anesthetic which also includes the mode of poisoning.

Be careful when selecting either combination or multiple codes because you do not code them as related unless the doctor makes a statement that they are related. This is because a patient may have a condition that can be coded as associated or due to another condition, but may in their case not be related. For example, a patient may be seen for treatment of cataracts and the patient has diabetes, but the two are not related and the cataracts are not caused by the diabetes. Therefore, the healthcare provider must clearly state that they are connected; otherwise, you would code them separately as having no relationship to each other.

Section 5.5: SEQUENCING

The linking of ICD-10-CM codes to CPT and HCPCS code is critical in physician coding. This will be discussed further in the CPT section. Sequencing is based on several formats:

First, sequencing is required when the ICD-10-CM book directs you to code a certain code first. Information regarding sequencing can be found in the coding guidelines in the front of the book which are very helpful when coding either on the job or during a test.

Sequencing can also be determined by determining which condition is the etiology and which is the manifestation. A manifestation is a condition that results from another condition known as the etiology. The etiology is the original condition that caused the manifestation. In these scenarios, the etiology is usually listed first. Oftentimes this will be denoted by explanatory notes within the codes, such as "code first" which is usually listed in the etiology code descriptions. For manifestation codes, there is usually a description of "code also" meaning that the etiology code should also be listed. In the alphabetical index this sequencing is denoted by the etiology code listed first and the manifestation code listed after in square brackets.

Second, the concept of sequencing is that the code for the main reason the patient received services is usually listed first.

Section 5.6: COMORBIDITIES/COMPLICATIONS

Comorbidities are conditions that are oftentimes associated with another condition and complications are conditions that can result from a condition. Although we do not always code conditions that exist at the time healthcare is provided for another condition, we do code them if they either receive treatment themselves or if they may influence the patient's care or the outcome and, therefore, MAY result in additional care and/or extended hospital stay which many comorbidities and complications do, such as diabetes or COPD.

With this definition, there are some comorbidities and complications that are typically coded in addition to the primary diagnosis for which the patient received care. These comorbidities and complications are coded also because either they require care for themselves or they are known to pose a great probability of affecting the outcome of the patient's care.

Probably the most familiar are diabetes and AIDS. These two conditions complicate most all other healthcare. For example, if a patient receives sutures for a minor wound, the diabetes may complicate things and result in longer healing and/or infection. Other conditions that are oftentimes coded in addition to the primary code are hypertension, heart problems, COPD and other breathing problems, and renal failure.

Section 5.7: SYMPTOMS

For physician coding, do not code symptoms if you have a diagnostic statement. Code only the diagnostic statement then such as diabetes, not the symptoms associated with it. Typically, with physician coding, you code the diagnostic statement and nothing else.

However, there are several scenarios in which you would code symptoms. First, this includes when no diagnostic statement is given or possible. This can occur because the symptoms are transient and were, therefore, not diagnosable. It can also occur if the tests are negative or abnormal but no definitive diagnosis is determined from it. If a physician is not able to conduct enough tests at the time of the visit, then he may not be able to determine the diagnosis. Cases may also be referred to another practice or hospital for determination of the diagnosis. You must code something and since you don't have a diagnostic statement, you will code the symptoms.

You would also code symptoms even if they are contained within the diagnosis code if they are being treated, such as a headache, fever, or dehydration.

Common symptoms may include fever, dehydration, headache, syncope, convulsions, dizziness, weakness, stomach ache, nausea, vomiting, diarrhea, urination problems, skin problems, palpitations, and breathing problems.

Section 5.8: RULE OUTS

Physician coding and hospital inpatient coding vary in many ways. One of the most prominent differences is that we never code diagnostic statements that contain "rule out," "possible," "probable", or any other term that is not a definite diagnosis for physician coding. This is because healthcare providers may not always have the time or ability to fully test and determine the cause of symptoms (the diagnosis), so we do not know if the "rule out" statement by a healthcare provider is true or not as opposed to the testing in the hospital which can be much longer and more intensive, therefore more defining and certain.

Remember, if a physician provides symptoms, and even if he uses a "rule out" diagnostic statement, we can only code the symptoms because **WE NEVER MAKE A DIAGNOSIS, so NOT DOCUMENTED, NOT DONE.** If you remember this critical coding rule, it will simplify your coding responsibilities and ensure correct coding. It is vital that you remember this because you can get into trouble if you start diagnosing the patient and use these codes to bill. It is a very serious situation in which a patient is given a diagnosis they do not have – this can have huge implication in many ways on their future care and may impact their lives in a myriad of ways. This serious situation is also complicated because once a patient is given a wrong diagnosis, that diagnosis becomes disseminated throughout a wide network of providers and organizations which makes it more difficult to remove and/or correct. In addition, the process to remove an incorrect diagnosis is extremely difficult and frustrating.
So, never code any diagnostic statement that does not clearly posit a diagnosis. Instead, you will have to code the symptoms.

If a condition is described as "borderline," code it as definitive unless there is a code that describes the condition as borderline in which case you would use that code.

Section 5.9: ACUTE/CHRONIC

Acute and chronic are definitions that come up repeatedly throughout the ICD-10 codes and will be discussed throughout the remainder of the packets in this course.

Acute means the condition has developed recently and is being treated at the present time. Chronic means that the condition has been ongoing in treatment over time. It is very important to distinguish between chronic and acute when coding because it makes a difference in several ways. The physician must describe it as chronic in order to be coded as chronic.

First, some codes do not distinguish between acute and chronic codes. If this is the case, the one code would be used for either one. If a condition is reported as both acute and chronic, but the code does not distinguish, you still only need to use the one code to describe both.

Second, some codes distinguish between acute and chronic codes. If this is the case, then you must select which code is accurate, either acute or chronic.

Third, some conditions may be both acute and chronic. A person may have a chronic condition which is present at the same time as the acute condition. In this case, you would have to code both acute and chronic, which again is reflected in the previously mentioned scenarios that you will use either one code that includes both acute and chronic or two separate codes, one for acute and one for chronic.

STRUCTURE QUIZ 1

1. What number most often represents an unspecified code?

2. What is the code for encephalopathy that is not specified?

3. Derangement of a previous ligament of the right knee is what code?

4. What are the codes for a perforation of the esophagus that was traumatic?

5. What number most often represents a code in which more information is provided but there is no specific code for the condition?

6. What is the code for spina bifida occulta?

7. What are the codes for otitis due to impetigo?

8. What are the codes for excessive vomiting in a pregnant woman?

9. What does NEC stand for?

10. What is the code for postviral encephalitis?

11. What is the code for a patient who is seen today for crushing chest injury?

12. A patient is seen today for a headache and polyneuropathy due to Type 1 diabetes. What are the codes?

13. A patient is seen today to rule out a hernia due to abdominal pain. What are the codes?

14. A patient is seen today for arthropathy due to TB of the hip. What are the codes?

15. A patient is seen today for a stomach ache and headache and was found to be due to botulism. What are the codes?

CHAPTER 6
ICD-10 INFECTIOUS DISEASES

You will learn the following objectives in this chapter:

A. Coding for Organisms
B. Infections
    1. Intestinal
    2. Tuberculosis
    3. Other
C. Sepsis
D. Sexually Transmitted
E. Viral
    1. Hepatitis
F. HIV/AIDS
G. Mycosis/Others
H. Sequelae

Section 6.1: CODING FOR ORGANISM

Chapter 1 is described as "Certain Infectious and Parasitic Diseases" and is coded as A00-B99. The term "certain' indicates that some related codes may be found in other sections, such as respiratory if related to colds or pneumonia. For example, tetanus during pregnancy may be found under code A34. HIV may be found under B20.

As with most of the codes in ICD-10, there is a much greater specificity and many conditions are now combined with the organism as one code, such as typhoid.

When coding for infectious and parasitic diseases be sure to use an additional code to identify the organism's resistance to antimicrobial drugs (Z16).

Remember, as with ICD-9, some conditions caused by an organism are included in the code for the organism. When coding for conditions caused by organisms, there are several coding scenarios that you may encounter so you must determine correct codes including those that involve multiple and combination coding.

When coding for conditions caused by an organism, you want to code the condition and the organism. If the organism is known and not included in a selected code, then a code from the section for infectious diseases needs to be coded also for the organism, such as B96.

One possible scenario in coding infectious diseases is combination coding scenarios in which one code can be found in the ICD-10 book which includes in its description both the condition and the organism.

If an organism is drug-resistant, this must also be coded such as with Z16, resistance to antimicrobial drugs as well as the combination code for the condition and the organism, such as MRSA, e.g. J15.212, if available. If there is not a combination code, then code the condition and organism separately. Sometimes a patient may be carrying a drug-resistant organism but display no symptoms. This is known as colonization and can be coded with Z22.322. If the patient is determined to be both carrying it and does have symptoms, then code both.

Organisms should always be coded, if known whether in a combination code or as an additional code to the condition. If not known, A41.9 could be used associated with sepsis.

INTESTINAL: Intestinal infectious diseases are coded as A00-A09. This includes typhoid, salmonella, shigellosis, and many others including food poisoning and dysentery.

Typhoid Fever (A01.0) and Amebic infections (A06.8) have a fifth character added which indicates site or type. Many other codes have been expanded to include manifestations such as Listeriosis (A32) and Whooping cough (A37).

TUBERCULOSIS: Tuberculosis is coded as A15-A19. While most TB codes are included in these codes, some are not, such as congenital TB which is coded as P37.0 which is in the congenital section of codes.

Tuberculosis can occur in various parts of the body such as nervous system, eyes, spine, intestines, and organs other than just the lungs. There are various related conditions that are now included in some TB codes such as arthritis.

A positive TB test but no symptoms is coded as R76.11 as noted under the exclude notes as well as other excluded conditions.

OTHER BACTERIAL INFECTIONS: A wide variety of bacterial conditions are coded from A20 to A38 such as the plague, anthrax, cat-scratch fever, meningitis, tetanus, staph, strep, whooping cough, and scarlet fever.

Leprosy (A30) has been expanded   with regards to type, e.g. Tuberculoid leprosy (A30.1) or lepromatous leprosy (A30.4).

Section 6.2: SEPSIS

There are various names used to refer to an infection caused by an organism within the human body. If allowed to grow, this infection can progress throughout the body and result in death. Although some of the terms used to denote this condition may be used interchangeably by healthcare providers, there are distinct differences within the terms and may involve the progression and severity of the infection within the body. If the infectious organism is not known, this is known as cryptogenic.

The progression of the infection is bacteremia to septicemia which is now known as sepsis to severe sepsis to severe sepsis with septic shock to multiple organ dysfunction to death. Sepsis is an infection. Urosepsis is a nonspecific term and should not be used. If used, the doctor should be queried as to whether this is sepsis or not. Puerperal sepsis refers to sepsis following childbirth. Cellulitis is infection of the skin. Lymphangitis is infection of the lymph glands.

Septicemia is when an organism has invaded the blood and is systemic. Forms of septicemia include bacteremia and sapremia. Bacteremia is when a bacteria has caused the infection and is further defined by the organism. Sapremia is when a toxin has caused the infection. Sepsis is coded from the other bacterial infection section and is specified by streptococcal (A40) and other (A41). Related septicemia and bacteremia are coded as R78.81.

There are several "code first" notes in this section for sepsis related to pregnancy, abortions, postprocedural, immunizations and infusions. There are also many "exclude" notes when sepsis is associated with specific organisms.

As sepsis continues, it can result in SIRS (systemic inflammatory response syndrome) which refers to an overwhelming septic infection and is coded with R65.1. Sometimes in the latter stages of infection, a physician may refer to the condition as severe sepsis which is coded as R65.2- with additional conditions listed after the code which denote what conditions make the sepsis qualify as severe. This includes shock and organ failure which would also be coded in addition to the sepsis code. The severe sepsis codes are now differentiated by the absence or presence of septic shock with R65.20 without and R65.21 with shock. Postprocedural septic shock is coded as T81.12.

Regarding sequencing, the underlying infection should be coded first and then the R65 codes for the sepsis. If the sepsis is due to a noninfectious process such as trauma, then code the trauma first.

Section 6.3: SEXUALLY TRANSMITTED

Codes A50-A64 include sexually transmitted diseases (STDs) other than AIDS which are highly differentiated such as whether they are congenital, late, early, secondary, symptomatic or asymptomatic and include related conditions such as endocarditis. This includes syphilis, gonococcal, chlamydia, and herpes, trichomoniasis.

OTHER: Other diseases include yaws, fevers, and lyme disease. There are also codes for rickettsiosis (A75-A79) which includes tick borne illnesses.

Section 6.4: VIRAL

Viral infections (A80-A89) include poliomyelitis, Creutzfeldt-Jakob disease, rabies, and mosquito-borne encephalitis. It also includes arthropod-borne viral diseases such as dengue fever, west nile, and yellow fever. Viral infections of the skin include herpes, chickenpox (varicella), smallpox, measles, rubella and viral warts.

HEPATITIS: Hepatitis is inflammation of the liver and can be viral or nonviral. Hepatitis codes are coded as being acute or chronic and if the delta-agent (Hepatitis D) is present with relationship to Hepatitis B.

There are several types of hepatitis.

Type A (B15) is highly contagious and usually transmitted fecally or orally. It was formerly known as infectious hepatitis and is the least serious form. Contaminated food is oftentimes the source and is typically spread under unsanitary conditions.

Type B (B16) is transmitted by contaminated blood, feces, and other human secretions. It was formerly known as serum hepatitis and is also known as chronic hepatitis. It can result in death from cirrhosis. It is transmitted by donated blood or serum transfusions, as well as sexually, which also includes dirty needles from drug use. The codes are differentiated by whether Hepatitis D and a coma are present.

Type C is usually transmitted by blood transfusions and use of dirty needles and sexual contact. C is the leading viral cause of chronic liver disease and can result in end-stage renal disease; however, some Type C hepatitis can be fulminating in that there is rapid onset.

Type D (also known as delta) is seen only in patients with Type B hepatitis because it cannot reproduce if the cell is not infected with Type B. Note that the fifth character also defines if Type D (delta) is mentioned.

Type E is transmitted enterally. Although not common in United States, it is common throughout the rest of the world due to infected water sources and causes epidemics.

These hepatitis codes also are further defined by whether there is a coma and if they are acute or chronic.

Other hepatitis include alcoholic, chemical, amebic, dirty needle, cholestatic, giant cell, interstitial, peliosis, posttransfusion, serum, syphillic, toxic, tuberculous, etc.

OTHER VIRAL: Other viral include CMV (B25), mumps (B26), infectious mononucleosis (B27) further specified by the type and the manifestation, conjunctivitis (B30) and numerous others.

Section 6.5: HIV/AIDS

There are some special coding circumstances surrounding the coding of HIV and AIDS. It is transmitted by sexual contact, body fluids, and dirty needles. There have been many misconceptions and limited information about HIV. There are two types of HIV: HIV-1 and HIV-2. It is HIV-1 that is known to cause AIDS

HIV (human immunodeficiency virus) means that the person has tested positive for the organism (a retrovirus) but may not have experienced any symptoms yet, so they are not considered to have the disease, AIDS (acquired immunodeficiency syndrome). AIDS is now pandemic in that it is an epidemic that has spread throughout various parts of the world. Most cases are in Africa.

HIV is coded as B20. If a patient has demonstrated symptoms due to HIV, then they are coded as having AIDS or symptomatic HIV disease using the code B20.

The manifestations should also be coded, that is what condition or symptoms the patient is experiencing that has resulted from the HIV virus. For example, if a patient has Kaposi's sarcoma due to HIV, then the person has the disease, AIDS, which would be listed first and the sarcoma second. HIV disease resulting in multiple infections in addition to the other conditions, B37.0 Candidal stomatitis, B37.1 Pulmonary candidiasis, and J99 respiratory disorders in other diseases specified elsewhere.

The B20 code should always be coded first, and any related conditions second. However, if a patient is seen for a condition, such as a fractured leg that is unrelated to the AIDS/HIV, then the condition would be listed first, and the AIDS/HIV second.

If the patient has tested positive for HIV, but has demonstrated no symptoms, then the correct code for their condition is Z21, asymptomatic HIV. If a patient is admitted for AIDS testing but there is no definitive positive diagnosis of HIV or AIDS, then code Z11.4.

If the patient is pregnant and is admitted for AIDS related condition, then code O98.7- followed by B20 as well as the related condition. If the HIV is asymptomatic in a pregnant patient, then code as O98.7- and Z21.

Once a patient is coded as B20 due to having manifestations of AIDS at some time, then they are always coded as B20 and never again as Z21.

If a patient's test has been inconclusive for HIV, then the correct code would be R75. If the results were negative, code Z71.7.

Section 6.6: MYCOSIS

Mycosis are fungal infections and can occur in various tissues such as different parts of the skin on different parts of the body (e.g. tinea pedis of the feet B35.3), candidiasis of various anatomic sites (B37), coccidiodomycosis (B38), histoplasmosis (B39), aspergillosis (B44), and cryptococcosis (B45).

OTHERS: Protozoal diseases (B50-B64) include malaria further specified by type and complications, e.g. plasmodium vivax malaria with rupture of spleen (B51.0). It also includes Chagas disease (B57), leishmaniasis (B55) and toxoplasmosis (B58). Helminthiasis (B65-B83) include schistosomiasis, flukes, taeniasis, filiariasis, hookworm, and enterobiasis. Pediculosis, acariasis, and other infestations are coded as B85-B89. Scabies is a parasitic infection of the skin characterized by pruritus. Tinea (ringworm) is a fungal infection of the skin, such as tinea corporis (ringworm) and tinea pedis (athlete's foot).

Section 6.7: SEQUELAE: Codes for sequelae of infections and parasitic disease are found at the end of the Chapter for infectious diseases (B90-B94).

INFECTIOUS DISEASES QUIZ 2

1. Is AIDS pandemic or epidemic?

2. What are the codes for septicemia due to anthrax?

3. What are the codes for a patient seen today for septic urinary tract infection due to E. coli?

4. What are the codes for a patient seen with hepatitis D associated with Hepatitis B?

5. What are the codes for a patient with uveitis due to syphilis?

6. What are the codes for a patient who has H. influenza due to meningitis?

7. What are the codes for a patient who has infection of the colon due to Clostridium difficile?

8. What are the codes for a patient seen today for HIV and related Kaposi's sarcoma of the lymph nodes?

9. What are the codes for a patient seen today with HIV?

10. What are the codes for chronic spondylitis?

11. What are the codes for a patient seen today for bacteremia with septic shock?

12. What are the codes for a patient with acute bronchitis due to Pseudomonas?

13. What are the codes for a patient with pernicious complications with nephropathy?

14. What are the codes for a patient seen today for SIRS with septic shock?

15. What are the codes for a 23-year-old patient who is seen today for MRSA?

CHAPTER 7
ICD-10 NEOPLASMS

You will learn the following in this chapter:

- A. Types of Neoplasms
    1. Benign neoplasm
    2. Uncertain behavior
    3. Unspecified behavior
    4. Malignant neoplasm
        a. In situ
        b. Primary/Secondary
- B. Grading and staging systems
    1. Grades
    2. TNM
- C. Location
- D. Alphabetical Index
- E. Sites
    1. Overlapping
    2. Multiple
    3. No Specification
- F. Chemotherapy/Follow-Up
- G. Neoplasm Table
- H. Complications
- I. Excision/History

Section 7.1: TYPES OF NEOPLASMS

A neoplasm is a growth (tumor) and can be benign, malignant, in situ, unspecified, or unknown as listed in the table. They are located in the second chapter of the Tabular Index with codes ranging from C00-D49. If your book is designed as such, please note that the indentation or color coding of the outer edges of the book designate the neoplasm section.

BENIGN NEOPLASM: A benign neoplasm is not cancerous (or bad) or spreading. The suffix, -oma, refers to benign neoplasms. For example, an osteoma is a benign neoplasm of the bone. This includes moles, polyps, lipoma (fatty tumor), adenomas (tumor of a gland), myoma (tumor of the muscle), angiomas (blood or lymph tissue tumors), papilloma (papillary tumor), meningiomas (brain tumors), cyst, and fibroids.

Although benign neoplasms are not associated with the dangers of a malignant (or cancerous) tumor, they can still pose health problems due to the pressure or complicating conditions they may cause on vital organs or structures.

Some benign neoplasms can progress to malignancy which is why they are observed and tested over time.

UNCERTAIN BEHAVIOR: Neoplasm of uncertain behavior means that it could not be determined from the tests if the neoplasm was malignant or benign.

UNSPECIFIED BEHAVIOR: Neoplasms that are unspecified means that no information was provided in the report to determine if the neoplasm was benign or malignant.

MALIGNANT NEOPLASM: A malignant neoplasm is cancerous and the term, malignancy, refers to bad. There are many terms used to indicate malignancy which are oftentimes designated by the location of the cancer. Cancer can occur in several places at the same anatomic site, for example, cancer could be in the bone, tissue, or skin on the leg.

Sarcomas are malignant neoplasms of the connective tissue, such as bone, fat, muscle, and cartilage, plus others. Melanomas are cancer of the pigment producing cells called melanoctyes which appear on the skin. PSA (prostate specific antigen) is a tumor market measured in the blood which is elevated in men with prostate cancer.

Malignant neoplasms are further described as in situ, primary, or secondary.

IN SITU: If it is contained and not spreading, the malignant neoplasm is known as "in situ". This classification, "in situ" can only be used if the physician states the neoplasm is in situ. Additional terms that indicate "in situ" include non-infiltrating, non-invasive, intraepithelial, and pre-invasive carcinoma.

PRIMARY/SECONDARY: Primary or secondary cancerous neoplasm are indicated by terms such as infiltrating and invasive which indicate the cancer is spreading.

Primary malignant neoplasms are the originating site for the cancer. Secondary malignant neoplasms are the sites where the cancer spread to (or metastasized).

Sometimes physicians may use terms other than "metastasis" to denote the spreading of the primary neoplasm to other sites. When you are not certain of the use of the term metastatic, substitute "spread" and you will be able to understand the term better. These terms include "spreading to/from" or "invasion to/from". Note the difference in the use of "to" or "from" and its relationship to either primary or secondary as the type of cancer. For example, if the physician states the liver cancer was metastatic or spreading from the breast, then it means the primary site was the breast and the liver cancer was the secondary site. If the physician states the colon cancer was metastatic or spreading to the bone, then the colon cancer was the primary site and the bone cancer was the secondary site.

There are some areas that are considered to be secondary if the morphology is not stated as to whether it is primary or secondary. These include:

Bone
Brain
Heart
Diaphragm
Liver
Lymph nodes
Mediastinum
Meninges
Peritoneum
Pleura
Retroperitoneum
Spinal Cord

Section 7.2: GRADE/STAGING

Grades are the degree of maturity or differentiation of the malignancy and are oftentimes used in assessing the prognosis for cancers, for example with PAP tests. There are four grades. Grade I are well differentiated tumors so they resemble their parent cell closely. This differentiation continues to decline as you progress through the other grades, from II to III and then finally to IV which carries the poorest prognosis.

TNM: TNM is the system used for staging. Staging is the extent of the malignancy's metastasis within the body.   T refers to the size and degree of the malignancy; N refers to the number of regional lymph nodes involved, and M refers to metastasis. The numbers range from 0 to 4 with 0 being the least (undetectable) and 4 being the most advanced. T stages range from 1 to 4; N stages range from 0 to 3; and M stages range from 0 to 1. Therefore, a malignancy might be coded as T1, N2, M1 which indicates the tumor is less than 3 cm in diameter (T1), metastasis to the lymph nodes in the trachea area (N3), and distant metastasis present (M1).

Section 7.3: LOCATION

Codes are differentiated initially by anatomic site. It is important to note that a neoplasm can occur in several areas of the same location on the body, so you must be careful that you code it correctly. For example, a neoplasm can occur in the skin, muscle, organ, bone, or other structure at the same anatomical site, such as the knee. Sometimes the neoplastic terms will indicate the specific location, such as sarcoma which indicates cancer of the skin or osteosarcoma which is cancer of the bone.

Section 7.4: ALPHABETICAL INDEX

If you are feeling confused by all of the various names for the many types of cancer and are wondering how you can embrace all of this, the alphabetical index is very helpful.   If you do not know what the terms mean that a physician uses to describe a neoplasm, you can simply look it up in the alphabetical index, and it will tell you what the neoplasm is, whether it is benign or malignant and what type it is with reference to its location. If the index lists it as being one or the other because some tumors can occur as malignant or benign, then you know what type of code to select. However, if the index lists the neoplasm as being either, then you must search the medical report to find out if it is malignant or benign.

Second, when the alphabetical index provides specific codes for a site under the tumor's name, such as leiomyoma of the uterus, you can simply use that code.

Third, if the alphabetical index does not provide a specific code under the term, then you must reference the neoplasm table as indicated in the alphabetical index.

Section 7.5: SITES

OVERLAPPING SITES:

The character 8 is oftentimes used in the fourth character to indicate that the neoplasm has spread to other contiguous or overlapping sites, e.g. C15.8 says "overlapping lesion of esophagus". If the site of origin is not known and the neoplasm is overlapping, there are also codes used to indicate this, e.g. C26.9 overlapping lesion of digestive system.

NO SPECIFICATION OF SITE: If no site is specified for the malignant neoplasm, then code C80, "Malignant neoplasm without specification of site", should be listed which can be used for primary or secondary sites.

Section 7.6: CHEMOTHERAPY/FOLLOW-UP

Remember in the ICD-9 book the V codes have codes for chemotherapy and follow-up exams. In ICD-10, those codes change to Z08.0 for follow-up exam (remember, a follow-up exam can only be coded as follow-up if treatment for the original condition has been completed as determined by the physician). Code Z51.1 is for chemotherapy and should be coded first if this is the reason the patient is seen. Personal history code for neoplasms are coded as Z85 codes.

If there is organ removal for prophylactic treatment of cancer, it would be coded as Z40.0. Z12 is for visits in which there is screening for cancer.

OTHER: The codes for malignant neoplasm of the esophagus (C15) has been changed from the ICD-9 in that reference to cervical, thoracic and abdominal has been eliminated. For other neoplasms, there has been an expansion of the codes by site, such as carcinoma in situ of skin, e.g. carcinoma in situ of skin or right eyelid, including canthus (D04.11).

There are new notes that direct the additional coding of factors that may have influenced the condition, such as tobacco dependence (F17) and exposure to tobacco smoke in the perinatal period (P96.81).

Hodgkin's Disease (C81) has been expanded to include types and lymph node involvement.

Section 7.7: NEOPLASM TABLE

When you know what terms you are looking for in the Neoplasm Table, then you can go to the Table and find the correct code. The Neoplasm Table lists the codes according to the specific location. For example, if you are coding osteosarcoma of the elbow, when you look under sarcoma in the alphabetical index, it directs you to check in the neoplasm table under bone and malignant. Remember to follow the directions of the alphabetical index precisely! Be sure to look under bone first, and not elbow. Once you have found bone in the neoplasm table, then you will look for elbow which has a code of C40.0.

> **VERY IMPORTANT! WHEN CODING FROM THE NEOPLASM TABLE AND ALPHABETICAL INDEX......BE SURE TO PICK THE CODE FROM THE CORRECT LINE**

Section 7.8: COMPLICATIONS

Complications should always be coded in addition to the neoplasm codes. Complications are sequences first if their treatment is the primary reason for the visit. Anemia is an exception in which the malignancy code would be listed first.

Section 7.9: EXCISIONS/HISTORY

If a malignancy has been removed, then it no longer exists. As long as the patient is treated for this malignancy, despite its removal, you will code the malignancy as existing. For example, if a patient has breast cancer and it is removed but the patient remains under chemotherapy for it and the physician does not describe the treatment as completed for the malignancy, then the code for breast cancer continues to be used. However, once the physician completes the treatment, then the breast cancer would be coded as a personal history of breast.

If a primary malignant neoplasm was removed but reoccurs at the same site then this should be coded as primary again.

NEOPLASMS QUIZ 3

1. What are the codes for intramural leiomyoma of the uterus?

2. What are the codes for a patient who is seen today for nausea and vomiting due to chemotherapy two days ago?

3. What are the codes for traumatic asphyxiation?

4. What are the codes for benign leiomyoma of the abdomen?

5. What are the codes for a patient who has metastatic brain cancer?

6. What are the codes for Paget's disease of the extramammary skin?

7. What are the codes for a patient with carcinoma of the body of the uterus and contiguous sites?

8. What are the codes for carcinoma of the rectum and colon metastatic from the anterior wall of the bladder?

9. What are the codes for adenoma of the chief cell?

10. What are the codes for a patient who is seen today for prophylactic chemotherapy a year after having a mastectomy due to breast cancer with treatment completed three months ago?

11. What are the codes for a patient who has Hodgkin's lymphoma of the lymph nodes of the neck and axilla and the spleen?

12. What are the codes for patient with malignant schwannoma of the abdomen?

13. What are the codes for leiomyoblastoma (include the M code) of the chest?

14. What are the codes for osteochondroma of the coccyx?

15. What are the codes for patient with UTI due to E. coli?

CHAPTER 8
ICD-10 BLOOD DISORDERS

You will learn the following objectives in this chapter:

A. Types of Blood Cells
B. Types of Blood Groups
C. RH Factor
D. Types of Blood Disorders
     1. Anemias
     2. Coagulation Defects
     3. Purpura/Hemorrhage
     4. White Blood Cell Disorders
     5. Other Diseases
E. Operative/Post Procedural
F. Immune Disorders
G. Leukemia
H. Multiple Myeloma

Chapter 3 is described as "Diseases of the Blood and Blood-forming Organs and Certain Disorders Involving the Immune Mechanism" and range from D50-D89. Some blood conditions are not coded in this chapter because other chapters have precedence over this chapter and so the blood condition may be coded in another chapter, such as neoplasms, pregnancy, perinatal, and organisms have a greater priority than the chapter for blood disorders for where conditions are coded, e.g. leukemia (cancer of the blood) are coded in Chapter 2, Neoplasms.

Section 8: TYPES OF BLOOD CELLS

Blood is composed of different types of cells. Erythrocytes are red blood cells. Leukocytes are white blood cells. There are five types of leukocytes: lymphocytes, basophils, eosinophils, neutrophils, and monocytes. Also known as thrombocytes, platelets are blood cells which are important in the process of blood clotting.

Section 8.2: TYPE OF BLOOD GROUPS

Blood groups are distinguished by the type of antigens and antibodies are present. The four blood types are:
     Type A contains A antigen and anti-B antibodies
     Type B contains B antigen and anti-A antibodies.
     Type AB contains both A and B antigens and no anti-A or anti-B antibodies.
     Type O contains no A or B antigens and both anti-A and anti-B antibodies.

The problem with donating blood is that if someone is Type B and they are given Type A, their anti-A antibodies will attack the blood which will result in hemolysis (breakdown of the blood) which can have serious consequences.

People with Type O blood are known as the universal donor because they have no A or B antigens so their blood can be accepted by anyone as there are no antigens to cause an attack by the antibodies. However, because Type O contains both types of antibodies, they cannot accept blood from anyone else except another Type O person.

Section 8.3: RH FACTOR

Rh factor is also an important issue with blood type, particularly with pregnancies. If a fetus is Rh+ (they have the Rh antigen), then their blood will incite the mother's blood to create antibodies to the Rh, so the first pregnancy does not pose any problems. The problem occurs when this mother gets pregnant again with another fetus that is Rh+ because now the mother's antibodies will attack the fetus' blood and destroy the Rh+ red blood cells. This condition is also known as erythroblastosis fetalis.

Section 8.4: ANEMIAS

Anemia is a deficiency in hemoglobin (a protein found inside red blood cells), either qualitative or quantitative. Hypoxia (lack of oxygen) occurs in anemia because sufficient blood with oxygen does not get to the cells. Anemia can result from several conditions, including hemorrhaging, iron deficiency, B12 deficiency (pernicious anemia), folic acid deficiency, hemolysis (red blood cell death), genetic (sickle cell anemia and thalassemia), nutritional deficiencies, and diseases.

The codes for anemia (D50-D64) have been expanded greatly to include more information about the type, e.g. thalassemia, beta type (D56.1). Secondary anemias are coded from D63 codes which are anemias due to other illness which will also need to be coded. If the anemia is drug-induced, there are coding notes that instruct the coding of E codes to identify the drug responsible. If caused by a poisoning, then the coding instruct that the substance should be coded first from T codes.

Nutritional anemias, such as iron deficiency anemia, are coded from D50-D53. Sickle cell anemia is coded as D57 and is subdivided by whether it is with or without crisis.

Sickle cell anemia is a genetic defect in which red blood cells exhibit a sickle shape resulting in severe hemolysis and pain, oftentimes resulting in death. With sickle cell anemia, there is a code for a person who has the genetic disease, but there is also a code for someone who is a carrier of the gene but does not have the symptoms. This is known as sickle cell trait (D57.3).

Hemolytic anemia (D59) is when the red blood cells are destroyed prematurely. It can be genetic or acquired (that is due to condition that occurs during a person's life). Acquired hemolytic anemia is broken into autoimmune and non-autoimmune. Non-autoimmune can be due to drugs, toxins, trauma, infections, liver disease, or septicemia. Autoimmune means the body is attacking the cells.

Aplastic anemia (D60) occurs when the bone marrow does not produce enough red blood cells. Included under this category of codes is pancytopenia which means deficiency in numbers of all cells, including red blood cells, white blood cells, and platelets.

Section 8.5: COAGULATION DEFECTS

Coagulation defects, purpura and other hemorrhagic conditions are coded as D65-D69. Other diseases are coded as D65-D69. Disorders involving the immune system are coded from D80-D89, such as sarcoidosis of lymph nodes (D86.1).

Coagulation is also known as blood clotting or the forming of a thrombus. Coagulation defects can occur due to genetic defects in clotting factors in the blood, synthesis problems, or breakdown of clotting factors. Vitamin K deficiency is one disorder that can result in coagulation defects. Hemophilia (D66) is a sex linked genetic recessive disorder in which a person bleeds easily and experiences difficulties in stopping the flow of blood due to the inability of the blood to clot. Bleeding can occur internally as well as externally. Von Willebrand disease (D68.0) is a genetic bleeding disorder in which a person bruises easily, has frequent nosebleeds, and has difficulty in profuse bleeding when cut, such as with surgeries.

Section 8.6: PURPURA/HEMORRHAGE

Hemorrhage is excessive bleeding. Purpura is red or purple colored discolorations of the skin caused by hemorrhaging. If the discolorations are smaller, they are known as petechiae and when they are larger they are known as ecchymoses. These conditions are frequently seen in thrombocytopenia (D69) which occurs when there is a low number of platelets in the blood.

Section 8.7: WHITE BLOOD CELL DISORDERS

Neutropenia (D70) is a reduction in circulating neutrophils which increases the risk of bacterial and fungal infections since the body does not have the means to fight the infections. Neutropenia occurs frequently in people receiving chemotherapy or other medications that suppress the immune system (D70.2). There are also codes for decreased or increased white blood cell count (D72).

Section 8.8: OTHER DISEASES

Other blood diseases include polycythemia (D75.1). This is an increase in the mass of the red blood cells or decrease in the volume of plasma and is measured in a lab as the hematocrit. Primary polycythemia can be caused by an abnormality of the bone marrow. Secondary polycythemia can be caused by heart or lung disease, smoking, renal or liver tumors, and endocrine abnormalities.

Section 8.9: OPERATIVE/POST PROCEDURAL

Hemorrhage and hematomas resulting from procedures are coded as D78.   Codes for the spleen have been expanded to include intraoperative and postprocedural complications (D78), e.g. accidental puncture or laceration during a procedure on the spleen (D78.1).

Section 8.10: IMMUNE DISORDERS

Immunodeficiencies other than AIDS are coded with D80-D89 codes. This includes hereditary, nonfamilial, antibody, selective, combined, variable and those with other major defects such as SCID (severe combined immunodeficiency), sarcoidosis, and graft-versus-host disease wherein the body reacts against grafts.

Section 8.11: LEUKEMIA

Leukemia is an increase in the cancerous white blood cells, but it is not coded from this section of the codes, but rather from the neoplasm chapter. Oftentimes treatment consist of chemotherapy and/or bone marrow transplants.

Section 8.12: MULTIPLE MYELOMA

Multiple myeloma is cancer of the bone marrow and is also coded in the neoplasm codes.

BLOOD DISORDERS QUIZ 4

1. What are the codes for a patient with senile dementia?

2. What are the codes for a patient experiencing septic shock due to UTI?

3. What are the codes for a patient suffering from dipsomania?

4. What are the codes for a patient with goat's milk anemia?

5. What are the codes for a patient who metastatic cancer of the uterus?

6. What are the codes for an anemic patient due to hemorrhaging of a lower leg wound caused by a car accident?

7. What are the codes for a patient who has sickle cell anemia Hb-SS with acute chest syndrome?

8. What are the codes for a patient who has vegan anemia?

9. What are the codes for a patient who has malignant schwannoma of the hip?

10. What are the codes for a patient experiencing a crisis with sickle cell anemia?

11. What are the codes for a patient who is diagnosed with anemia due to a chronic gastric ulcer?

12. What are the codes for a patient with Hodgkins lymphoma of the spleen and axillary and neck lymph nodes who has neutropenia due to chemotherapy?

13. What are the codes for a patient with traumatic asphyxiation?

14. What are the codes for a patient with a coagulation defect due to Vitamin K deficiency?

15. What are the codes for a patient who Pelger-Huet anomaly?

CHAPTER 9
ICD-10 ENDOCRINE

You will learn the following objectives in this chapter:

A. Endocrine System
B. Endocrine Glands
C. Diabetes
    1. Diabetes Mellitus
    2. Other
D. Operative Complications
E. Nutritional/Metabolic

Chapter 4 is described as "Endocrine, Nutritional and Metabolic Diseases" and range from E00-E89. There are many new subchapters in this Chapter including diabetes and malnutrition.

Section 9.1: ENDOCRINE SYSTEM

The endocrine system involves various glands within the body which secrete a large variety of hormones into the blood that control in many ways the vital functions of our body. In contrast, the exocrine system secrete their chemical substances into ducts and out of the body which include sweat, mammary, salivary, lacrimal (tear), and mucous glands.

Major endocrine glands include the hypothalamus, pituitary gland, pineal, thymus, parathyroids, pancreatic islets of Langerhans, thyroid, adrenals, ovaries, and testicles. The pituitary gland is known as the master gland as it controls most of the glandular activities. The endocrine section of the codes also includes nutritional, metabolic, and immunity disorders and diseases.

The pituitary gland is located in the brain and is also known as the hypophysis. It secretes a wide variety of hormones including the thyroid stimulating hormone and various growth hormones. Inadequate secretion of the growth hormones may result in hypopituitarism and dwarfism.

The thyroid glands secrete thyroxine (T4) and tri-iodothyronine (T3) which influences metabolism and control of the body temperature. A goiter of the thyroid may result which is enlargement of the thyroid gland due to hypoactivity or hyperactivity of the thyroid or a deficiency in iodine. Graves' disease may occur in hyperthyroidism. Hypothyroidism is known as myxedema and may result in mental retardation and dwarfism.

There are four parathyroid glands are located on the posterior sides of the thyroid glands. These glands regulate the calcium and phosphate in the body.

Adrenal glands are located above the kidneys. They secrete steroids which regulate salt balance, metabolism, and sex development (androgens and estrogen) as well as epinephrine, norepinephrine, cortisone and cortisol. Hyperadrenalism can result in Cushing's Syndrome or Addison's disease.

In the medical field, this is probably the most neglected field with large cities oftentimes only have a couple of physicians who specialize in this area; yet, this area of medicine is probably one of the most critical to our general health and is found to contribute significantly to many symptoms and conditions as evidenced by the rapid growth in autoimmune diseases and diabetes.

Various deficiencies can result from the failure of these glands which are aggravated by poor nutrition and exposure to toxins and can be due to trauma, tumors, surgery, radiation, or genetic defects. Deficiencies can result in the over or under production of hormones.

Section 9.2: ENDOCRINE GLANDS

Disorders of the thyroid gland are coded as E00-E07 including goiters, iodine-deficiency, thyrotoxicosis and thyroiditis. Disorders of other endocrine glands are coded as E20-E35, such as hypoparathyroidism, hypopituitarism, Cushing's syndrome, hyperaldosteronism, ovarian and testicular dysfunction.

Section 9.3: DIABETES

There are two types of diabetes: mellitus and insipidus. There are significant differences between the two types. Symptoms for both diabetes include polydipsia (excessive thirst) and polyuria (excessive urination), but there is also hyperglycemia (excessive sugar) and glycosuria (sugar in the urine) in diabetes mellitus. The presence of ketones and rapid weight loss may also indicate diabetes mellitus.

DIABETES MELLITUS: The most common type is diabetes mellitus which is caused by the improper secretion and utilization of insulin which is produced by the pancreas and, therefore, the body is not able to properly utilize sugar and instead excretes it in the urine. Diabetes mellitus can be controlled or uncontrolled.

There are two types of diabetes mellitus· Type I and Type II. Type II is the most common type and does not require insulin therapy; however, there may be times when this type of diabetes is treated with insulin; therefore, a person being on insulin does not necessarily mean they are Type I so the physician must describe if the diabetes is Type I or Type II. If not known, then it would be coded as Type II/unspecified.

Type I is known as juvenile type or insulin-dependent diabetes mellitus (IDDM) because it develops most often in childhood. In Type I there is a complete lack of insulin so Type I is treated with insulin through injections or orally with daily blood monitoring and diet.

The two major changes to the diabetes codes are there are now five categories for diabetes and manifestations and complications are now indicated by the fourth or fifth character so there is no need for additional codes for them.

Diabetes is coded in three levels as Type I insulin-dependent/juvenile (E10), Type II non-insulin-dependent (E11), and other specified (E13). If the type of diabetes is not specified, then it should be coded as Type II, even if they are given insulin. Type I or juvenile just be specified in order to code Type I.

There are also codes for secondary diabetes mellitus due to underlying conditions (E08) and due to drugs or chemicals (E09) in which the underlying condition should be coded first as directed by the coding notes.

There are then fourth character classifications by complications which are much more extensive than they were in the ICD-9 codes. A fourth character of 6 indicates that the complication is not listed in the previous classifications, so this is an "other" code. A fourth character of 7 indicates that there are multiple complications. A fourth character of 8 indicates complications were mentioned but not identified. A fourth character of 9 indicates there are no identified complications. Remember, if the complication is known, then it should also be coded, e.g. diabetic cataracts would be coded as E13.36 and then H28 for the diabetic cataracts whose positioning as second denoted by an asterisk. Be careful to assure that the physician has diagnosed the complication as being related to the diabetes in order to code them together. If the condition is not due to the diabetes, then do not code the complication as being due to the diabetes.

There are new codes for diabetes mellitus caused by drugs or chemicals (E09), e.g. drug or chemical induced diabetes mellitus with renal complications (E09.2).

There is also a note in these codes that directs the coding of long-term insulin use (Z79.4).

If there are complications due to an insulin pump, this should be coded as T85.614.

OTHER: Hypoglycemia is coded with E15 and E16 codes with many differentiations of codes based on related conditions.

Diabetes insipidus is caused by the body's failure to adequately utilize antidiuretic hormone (ADH) which results in the kidneys not being able to properly reabsorb water into the bloodstream. Because the water is not reabsorbed, it is excreted in urine which is why urine in diabetes insipidus is watery and tasteless.   In contrast, urine in diabetes mellitus is sweet due to the presence of excessive amounts of sugar which was not properly used by the body and, therefore, excreted in the urine. Diabetes insipidus can be treated by the administration of ADH either by injection or orally. Diabetes insipidus is coded with E23.2.

Gestational diabetes can occur when a woman is pregnant and is due to increased metabolic demands during this time, so a woman may be diagnosed with gestational diabetes who is not diabetic when not pregnant, but she does have the potential to become diabetic in the future if not treated. This is not coded in this section but is listed in the pregnancy chapter.

Section 9.4: OPERATIVE COMPLICATIONS:

Intraoperative or postprocedural complications are coded as E36 for complications of the endocrine system developed from a procedure, e.g. postprocedural hemorrhage of an endocrine organ following an endocrine procedure (E36.01). Postprocedural complications for endocrine and metabolic are coded as E89.

Section 9.5: NUTRITIONAL/METABOLIC

Malnutrition is coded with codes E40-E46. Other nutritional deficiencies (E50-E64) include deficiencies of various vitamins such as B12, thiamine, D, E, and K as well as nutrients such as copper, magnesium and iron.

Weight codes (E66-E68) include overweight, obesity, and hyperalimentation.

Metabolic disorders (E70-E88) include albinism, PKT, maple-syrup-urine disease, fatty acid metabolism, carnitine, glycoprotein, lipid storage, lactose intolerance, X-linked disorders, fructose intolerance, Cori disease, Niemann-Pick disease (Type A, B, C or D), uricemia, bilirubin, minerals, volume depletion, hyperkalemia, and fluid overload. Cystic fibrosis is coded as E84. Hypercholesterolemia and hyperlipidemia are coded as E78 codes. Dehydration is coded as E86.0.

ENDOCRINE QUIZ 5

1. What are the codes for a patient with drug-induced Cushing's syndrome?

2. What are the codes for a patient with H. influenza with meningitis?

3. What are the codes for a patient with anemia and ALS?

4. What are the codes for a patient with polyuria due to possible diabetes mellitus?

5. What are the codes for a Type I diabetic patient with cataracts?

6. What are the codes for a patient with arthritis due to chronic gout?

7. What are the codes for a patient with Hodgkins lymphoma of the spleen and axillary and neck lymph nodes?

8. What are the codes for a patient treated with insulin in the emergency room due to severe ketoacidosis due to their diabetes mellitus?

9. What are the codes for a patient who experienced hypovolemic shock due to trauma?

10. What are the codes for a patient with goiter related to hyperthyroidism with storm?

11. What are the codes for a patient with diabetic retinal microangiopathy with edema?

12. What are the codes for a patient with a headache and possible concussion?

13. What are the codes for hypopituitarism due to the administration of radiotherapy?

14. What are the codes for a patient experiencing a thyrotoxic crisis due to Graves' Disease?

15. What are the codes for a patient who has amputation of two toes on the right foot due to gangrene related to Type 2 diabetic peripheral vascular disease?

CHAPTER 10
ICD-10 MENTAL

You will learn the following objectives in this chapter:

A. DSM-IV-TR
B. Mental Disorders due to Physiological Conditions
C. Psychoactive Substances
D. Psychosis
E. Neurosis
F. Behavioral Syndromes
G. Disorders of Adult Personality
H. Intellectual Disabilities
I. Developmental Disorders
J. Childhood Disorders

Chapter 5 is described as "Mental and Behavioral Disorders" and range from F01-F99.

Section 13.1: DSM-IV-TR

Another form of coding used with mental disorders is the DSM-IV (Diagnostic and Statistical Manual of Mental Disorders, Fourth Edition, Text Revision) published by the American Psychiatric Association. It is composed of Axis I, Axis II, Axis III, Axis IV, and Axis V. Axis I is for Clinical Disorders and Other Conditions including all psychiatric disorders which are now described by the use of ICD-10 codes. Axis II contains the personality disorder and mental retardation classifications. Axis II contains the medical conditions. Axis IV contains psychological and environmental conditions that influence the care. Axis V contains the psychological, social,

Section 10.2: MENTAL DISORDERS DUE TO PHYSIOLOGICAL CONDITIONS

Mental disorders due to physiological conditions (F01-F09) (formerly described as organic) include mental conditions and disorders that developed due to an actual physical condition such as dementia, amnesia, delirium, hallucinations, catatonic, mood, personality, and behavioral which may be caused by conditions such as epilepsy, concussions, and Alzheimer's. Dementia is the loss or impairment of thinking and distinguished as senile or presenile with other conditions such as delirium, delusions, and depression. Senile dementia is dementia occurring in people over the age of 65. Presenile dementia is dementia occurring in people younger than 65 years of age. The same codes are now used for both senile and presenile (F03). Delirium is acute temporary disturbance of consciousness in which a patient may be incoherent and disoriented.

Mental conditions due to alcohol or drugs are excluded from this section and are coded with F10-F19.

Section 10.3: PSYCHOACTIVE SUBSTANCES

Disorders due to psychoactive substances, such as alcohol, opioids, cocaine, and tobacco are coded with codes F10-F19. The fourth character specifies the clinical state as .0 acute intoxication; .1 harmful use; .2 dependence syndrome; .3 withdrawal state; .4 withdrawal state with delirium; .5 psychotic disorder; .6 amnesiac disorder; .7 residual and late-onset psychotic disorder; .8 other; and .9 unspecified. Fifth and sixth characters provide greater specificity about complications, such as sleep disturbance or delusions.

There are notes indicating that an additional code needs to be listed for blood alcohol level (Y90).

There is greater emphasis on nicotine use which is coded with F17 codes.

Alcoholism denotes an ongoing long-term abuse of alcohol in which a person mentally and physically has become dependent on alcohol as defined by the doctor, therefore it is described as a dependence. Continuous refers to regular ingestion of large amounts of alcohol, usually daily or weekly. Episodic refers to alcoholic binges which can last weeks or months which can be followed by periods of sobriety. In remission means that the patient is no longer consuming alcoholism or is in the process of significant reduction in their consumptions. However, once a person is diagnosed with dependence, they are treated as having dependence for life although it may be in remission because any encounter with alcohol can result in the return of their mental and physical dependencies. With alcoholism there may be other conditions that also need to be coded such as cirrhosis or hepatitis since alcoholism damages the health of a patient in many ways. Acute alcohol abuse refers to a one time abuse of alcohol which may occur in someone who is either dependent or not dependent on alcohol.

Section 10.4: PSYCHOSIS

Codes F20-F29 describe more serious psychosis including schizophrenia, bipolar disorder, and manic depressive disorder.

Schizophrenia (F20) is characterized by disturbances in thinking, mood and behavior with an altered concept of reality with possible hallucinations and delusions. Schizophrenia is classified by type: simple, disorganized, catatonic, paranoid, schizophreniform, latent, residual, schizoaffective, other, and unspecified. In catatonic schizophrenia, the patient is unresponsive and characterized by rigid positioning. Disorganized schizophrenia includes a lack of ability to associate with rapid shifting between thoughts so that the patient appears incoherent. In paranoid schizophrenia, the person imagines feelings of grandeur or persecution. Schizoaffective disorder (F25) is schizophrenia combined with affective mood disorders.

Affective mood disorders (F30-F39) are characterized by mood disturbances, such as manic, depressive, and bipolar. Mood disorder codes have been expanded to further describe the severity of bipolar disease (manic episode), e.g. manic episode without psychotic symptoms, mild (F30.11). Other nonpsychotic disorders have also been expanded through the use of fourth, fifth and sixth characters, e.g. blood, injection, injury type phobia, fear of other medical care

(F40.232).

Bipolar disorder (F31) is a mood disorder in which a person experiences rapid mood swings from manic levels of high to lows, known as mania and depression. Bipolar I are manic episodes with some depressive episodes, while Bipolar II is primarily depressive episodes marked by some periods of high manic behavior. Cyclothymia is a milder form of bipolar disorder. Major depression (F32) can be mild, moderate or severe with or without psychotic features and as a single episode or recurrent.

Depression can be major involving long continuous periods of depression marked by the patient's belief that the depression will not end. Dysthymia (F34.1) is a less severe form of depression that does not typically last as long and does not involved psychotic features such as hallucinations and paranoia.

Section 10.5: NEUROSIS

These codes (F40-F48) describe less severe mental conditions known as neurosis or personality disorders, in other words "nonpsychotic". This includes anxiety disorders, panic disorder, hysteria, phobias, histrionic and schizoid personality disorders, gender disorders, eating disorders, adjustment reaction, autism, sleep disorders, depression, speech and language disorders, conduct disorders, hyperactivity, and drug problems. Histrionic is when a patient is emotional and attention-seeking characterized by outbursts and tantrums. Schizoid is when the patient is cold and indifferent to other's emotions.

Anxiety disorders are coded with F40 codes, such as phobias like agoraphobia. Phobias are when a person has a great fear of something to the point of irrationality and debilitation. Phobias include agoraphobia which is a fear of being out in public. Social anxiety disorder is a phobia of social interaction. Claustrophobia is a fear of closed-in areas. Acrophobia is a fear of heights.

Other anxiety disorders include panic attacks (F41.0). Obsessive-compulsive disorder is coded as F42. Obsessive-compulsive disorders are when a person experiences recurrent thoughts and experience a dominant need to perform repeated acts. Obsessive-compulsive disorder is not coded the same as obsessive-compulsive personality disorder (F60.5) because it is not a personality disorder.

Dissociative disorders are when a patient has impairment of perception and consciousness and can include split personalities which can be a means of compensation for trauma or conflicts.

Another condition that develops from the attempt to compensate for past trauma is post traumatic stress disorder. Reaction to severe stress is coded as F43 such as post traumatic stress disorder (PTSD) which is coded as F43.1.

Adjustment disorders are coded as F43.2. Dissociative and conversion disorders are coded as F44 which include fugues, stupors, seizures, convulsions and motor symptoms related to the disorder.

Somatoform disorders (F45) are disorders which are evidenced in physical symptoms. This includes hypochondriasis which is an abnormal preoccupation with illnesses and physical problems. In a conversion disorder the patient experiences loss of physical functions based on their fear.

Section 10.6: BEHAVIORAL SYNDROMES ASSOCIATED WITH PHYSIOLOGICAL DISTURBANCES

There are several behavioral syndromes with physiological disturbances (F50-F59) that can occur. Eating Disorders (F50) include bulima nervosa, anorexia nervosa, pica, and rumination. Bulima is binge eating followed by self-induced vomiting. Anorexia nervosa is the failure to eat sufficient food to sustain life as evidenced by severe weight loss and a development of many other life-threatening conditions. Pica is the eating of inedible substances. Rumination is the regurgitation and re-swallowing of food, which is typically described as occurring in cows but is performed by some people.

Sleep disturbances (F51) include insomnia, hypersomnia, sleepwalking, nightmares, and sleep terrors.

Sexual dysfunctions (F52) include hypoactive sexual desire, sexual aversion, and sexual arousal disorders as well as orgasmic disorders. Postpartum depression is coded as F53.

Abuse of non-psychotic substances (F55) include abuse of antacids, laxatives, steroids, and vitamins.

Section 10.7: DISORDERS OF ADULT PERSONALITY

Disorders of adult personality and behavior (F60-F69) include paranoid, antisocial, borderline, histrionic, obsessive-compulsive, avoidant, and dependent. Impulse disorders (F63) include pathological gambling, pyromania, kleptomania, and trichotillomania (hair plucking). Gender identity disorders are coded as F64. Various paraphilias (F65) include fetishism, pedophilia, sadomasochism, necrophilia, and voyeurism.

Section 10.8: INTELLECTUAL DISABILITIES

Intellectual disabilities (F70-F79) include mental retardation which is coded as mild (F70), moderate (F71), severe (F72), profound (F73), other (F78) and unspecified (F79). Impairment of behavior is coded in the fourth character as .0 for no or minimal impairment of behavior, .1 for significant impairment, .8 for other impairments, and .9 for no mention of impairment. Notice that .0 is for when there is a statement that there is no or minimal impairment, but .9 is when there is no mention.

Section 10.9: DEVELOPMENTAL DISORDERS

Pervasive and specific developmental disorders (F80-F89) include disorders with language, speech, scholastic (reading and math), writing, learning disabilities, and clumsy child. Autism (F84.0) is also included as well as Rett's syndrome and Asperger's syndrome.

Section 10.10: BEHAVIORAL AND EMOTIONAL DISORDERS IN CHILDHOOD

Behavioral and emotional disorders with onset usually occurring in childhood and adolescence (F90-F98) may be used regardless of the patient's age as long as the disorder developing during childhood or adolescence. These codes include attention deficit hyperactivity disorder, conduct disorders, separation anxiety, selective mutism, reactive attachment disorder, tic disorders (Tourette's and motor), enuresis, encopresis, feeding disorders, pica, thumb-sucking, and nail-biting.

MENTAL QUIZ 6

1. What are the codes for a patient with carcinoma of the lower outer quadrant of the breast metastatic to the left lung?

2. What are the codes for patient experiencing panic attack with agoraphobia?

3. What are the codes for a patient who is experiencing combat fatigue?

4. What are the codes for a patient who has chronic alcoholism with cirrhosis?

5. What are the codes for a patient with anorexia?

6. What are the codes for a patient suffering from depression due to the death of her husband?

7. What are the codes for a teenager who has been experiencing problems with significant school truancy?

8. What are the codes for a patient with subacute borderline schizophrenia?

9. What are the codes for a patient with a long history of alcoholism who was binge drinking over the superbowl weekend and seen for drunkenness?

10. What are the codes for a patient with dementia due to alcohol intoxication?

11. What are the codes for a 62-year-old patient with paranoid senile dementia?

12. What are the codes for a patient with bulima nervosa?

13. What are the codes for a patient with chronic PTSD?

14. What are the codes for a patient who has an IQ of 65?

15. What are the codes for a patient with acute exacerbation of chronic myeloid leukemia?

CHAPTER 11
ICD-10 NERVOUS SYSTEM

You will learn the following in this chapter:

A. Nervous System
    1. Central Nervous System
    2. Peripheral Nervous System
B. Inflammatory Conditions
    1. Meningitis
    2. Encephalitis
    3. Myelitis
C. Movement Disorders
    1. Systemic Atrophies
    2. Extrapyramidal
    3. Degenerative
D. Epilepsy
E. Migraines/Headaches
F. Nerve Disorders
G. Cerebral Palsy/Paralytic Syndromes
H. Other Disorders
I. Procedural Complications

Chapter 6 is described as "Diseases of the Nervous System" and range from G00-G99. Most of these codes are secondary codes because many of these conditions are listed in other chapters, such as perinatal, pregnancy, neoplasms, and injuries.

Section 11.1: NERVOUS SYSTEM

The codes relating to the nervous system include the central nervous system and the peripheral nervous system. Remember, these codes refer to the nervous system and not the bones of the spinal cord which are included in the musculoskeletal section of the codes.

The central nervous system (CNS) includes the brain and the spinal cord. The brain is surrounded by three layers of connective tissue known as the meninges. The outermost layer is known as dura mater, the second layer is known as arachnoid membrane, and the third layer is pia mater. Between the first and second layer is the subdural space and between the second and third there is a space called subarachnoid space.

The peripheral nervous system (PNS) consists of 11 pairs of cranial nerves (cranial nerve II is not included in the PNS) outside of the brain and spinal cord. They carry impulses throughout the rest of the body. Peripheral nerves carry impulses from the CNS to nerves that function involuntarily or voluntarily. The autonomic nervous system (ANS) is a part of the PNS which can be enteric, sympathethic or parasympathetic. The sympathetic and parasympathetic react in opposite ways to each other to either increase or decrease body functions such as fight or flight response which increases blood pressure from the sympathetic opposite to the parasympathetic response of reducing blood pressure. The enteric influences the GI tract. There is a fluid that circulates throughout the brain and spinal cord which provides a cushion to prevent shock and is known as cerebrospinal fluid (CSF).

Section 11.2: INFLAMMATORY CONDITIONS

Meningitis is coded as G00-G04. Meningitis is the inflammation of the meninges that surround the brain and is caused by microorganisms. The organism is now included in the meningitis code such as bacterial or other.

Encephalitis (G04) is the inflammation of the brain, which derives from the term encephalo. Myelitis is the inflammation of the spinal cord. Encephalomyelitis is inflammation of the brain and spinal cord. Intracranial and intraspinal abscess and granulomas are coded as G06 or as in other diseases (G07). Intracranial and intraspinal phlebitis and thrombophlebitis is coded as G08.

Sequelae of inflammatory disease of the CNS are coded as G09.

Section 11.3: MOVEMENT DISORDERS

SYSTEMIC ATROPHIES: Systemic atrophies primarily affecting the central nervous system (CNS) (G10-G14) include Huntington disease coded as G10. These codes also include hereditary ataxia such as cerebellar, spinal muscular atrophy, and atrophies affecting the CNS in other diseases. Postpolio syndrome (G14) is also included.

EXTRAPYRAMIDAL AND MOVEMENT DISORDERS: Extrapyramidal and movement disorders (G20-G26) include Parkinson's disease coded as G20-G26 and has been expanded to include type. Parkinson's disease due to other conditions is coded as G21. Other disorders include dystonia which can be drug induced, genetic torsion, tremors, myoclonus, chorea, tics restless leg syndrome, and stiff-man syndrome with many differentiated by whether they are drug induced or not.

OTHER DEGENERATIVE DISEASES: Alzheimer's disease is coded as G30 which is further specified by age at onset, either early or late. Other degenerative disorders include Pick's disease and degeneration with separate codes for drug induced.

DEMYELINATING DISEASES: Demyelinating diseases of the CNS (G35-G37) include multiple sclerosis. Other diseases include demyelinations such as of the central pontine or myelitis.

Section 11.4: EPILEPSY

Grand mal seizures, also known as generalized tonic-clonic seizures, are characterized by involvement of the entire body including muscle rigidity, muscle contractions, and loss of consciousness. In the tonic phase, the muscles tighten up and in the clonic phase the muscles experience spasms. Petit mal seizures, also known as absence seizures, are characterized by a very short loss of consciousness and functions demonstrated by an absent look with or without twitching movements of muscles. Idiopathic epilepsy means the cause is not known.

Epilepsy is coded as G40 and is further specified by the type of seizure and epilepsy (localized, idiopathic, generalized, petit mal and grand mal) as well as types of seizures, if intractable and with or without status epilepticus. Epilepsy is a paroxysmal disorder characterized by recurrent seizures. The codes are differentiated by the terms generalized, complete partial, or simple partial. In a partial seizure, the disturbance is limited to a specific area of the brain as opposed to generalized which is not specific in area. Generalized codes are further classified by intractable or not intractable (intractable means not responding to treatment), and with or without status epilepticus. There are codes for drug-induced epilepsy (G40.5). There are also codes for absence epileptic syndrome (G40.A) and Juvenile (G40.B). Other epileptic codes include Lennox-gastaut syndrome (G40.81) and spasms (G40.82).

Grand mal and petite male seizures are no longer differentiated and are coded as G40.4, generalized epilepsy NEC.

Section 11.5: MIGRAINES/HEADACHES

Migraines are coded as G43 and have been expanded to fifth characters to indicate the presence of status migrainosus. If drugs are involved, then the drug needs to be identified using T codes. Migraines are differentiated as with or without auras and intractable or not intractable. Other types of migraines include hemiplegic, persistent with or without cerebral infarction, chronic (G43.7), cyclical vomiting, ophthalmoplegic, periodic, abdominal, and menstrual.

General description of headache is coded as R51. However, this section of the codes include some types of headaches (G44) which include cluster headaches, vascular, tension, post-traumatic, and drug-induced.

Sleep disorders (G47) include insomnia other than due to alcohol or drugs as well as other exclusions as noted in the chapter on mental disorders. Hypersomnia, circadian rhythm sleep disorders, apnea, narcolepsy, cataplexy, parasomnia, and bruxism are included in this section too.

Section 11.6: NERVE DISORDERS

Nerve, nerve root and plexus disorders (G50-G59) include disorders of the various nerves such as the trigeminal, facial, cranial, and brachial plexus. Bell's palsy is coded as G51.0. Phantom limb (G54.6) syndrome is now differentiated as to whether pain is present or not.

Mononeuropathies (G56) include carpal tunnel syndrome and other lesions/causalgias of various nerves of the limbs, both arms and legs.

Polyneuropathies are coded as G60-G65 and can be hereditary, idiopathic, inflammatory, drug-induced, radiation-induced, or due to diseases. Sequelae of polyneuropathies are coded as G65.

Myoneural disease (G70-G73) include myasthenia gravis, muscular dystrophy (G71.0), myotonic disorders, and congenital myopathies. Myopathies (G72) can also be drug-induced, alcoholic, inflammatory, critical illness, or due to toxic agents.

Section 11.7: CEREBRAL PALSY & PARALYTIC SYNDROMES

Cerebral palsy and other paralytic syndromes are coded as G80-G83. Cerebral palsy (G80) can be spastic, quadriplegic, diplegic, hemiplegic, ataxis, or athetoid. Spastic includes congenital that develops when a child is young and is a result of brain damage from birth trauma or intrauterine pathology. Cerebral palsy refers to various disorders within the development of muscles and their coordination so it affects body movement, posture, and balance. Paralysis, such as quadriplegia and hemiplegia, are common as well as muscle stiffness and poor tone, uncontrolled movements, mental retardation, skeletal deformities, problems with speech and swallowing, and many more.

Hemiplegia and hemiparesis (G81) both mean paralysis of one side of the body but hemiparesis is less severe as it is weakness rather than complete paralysis. These codes are differentiated as to whether they are flaccid, spastic, other, or unspecified. Flaccid is loss of muscle tone. Spastic means rigidity of paralysis in combination with muscular contractions or spasms. The fifth character specifies if the paralysis is affecting the dominant or nondominant side of the body. Dominant side means if they are right-handed, the right side is dominant and the left side is non-dominant. If they are left-handed, the left side is dominant and the right side is non-dominant. Remember from anatomy and physiology that there is a cross-over between the brain and the body, so if the right side of the brain was damaged, then the left side of the body is affected and vice versa for damage to the left side of the brain. Remember though, the physician needs to document this. If none of this information is provided, then you must use the unspecified code.

Other kinds of plegia (G82) include quadriplegia which means complete paralysis of the body from the neck down and is also known as tetraplegia. Paraplegia refers to complete paralysis from the waist down. For quadriplegia the exact cervical location of the damage to the spine must be specified. These are further defined as complete or incomplete. While complete refers to complete loss of sensory or motor function below where the spinal cord injury occurred, incomplete indicates that there is some sensory or motor function below the injury site.

Monoplegia (G83) are described as to location, such as limbs and dominant or non-dominant side.

Section 11.8: OTHER DISORDERS

Other disorders of the nervous system (G89-G99) include pain which has many exclude notes. It can be differentiated as to acute or chronic and due to trauma or post-procedural. Chronic pain syndrome is coded as G89.4.

Other disorders include autonomic dysreflexia, complex regional pain syndrome (CRPS), hydrocephalus, encephalopathy, cerebral cysts, anoxic brain damage excluding that due to anesthesia or neonatal, compression of brain, brain death, cord compression, and cerebrospinal fluid leak.

Section 11.9: PROCEDURAL COMPLICATIONS

Intraoperative and postprocedural complications of the nervous system are coded as G97 including hypotension, puncture, laceration, hemorrhage and hematoma.

NERVOUS QUIZ 7

1. What are the codes for a patient with a classic migraine with aura?

2. What are the codes for a patient with an IQ of 45 who has ringworm?

3. What are the codes for a patient who has MS?

4. What are the codes for a patient who has pars planitis?

5. What are the codes for a patient who has double vision?

6. What are the codes for a patient who has pigmentary open-angle glaucoma?

7. What are the codes for a patient who has Fusarium keratitis?

8. What are the codes for a patient who has tonic-clonic epilepsy?

9. What are the codes for a patient who has restless leg syndrome?

10. What are the codes for a patient who presents today because she has not been taking her insulin as prescribed for her for the past four years and she is now experiencing polyneuropathy due to Type 2 diabetes?

11. What are the codes for a patient who has presenile cortical cataract of the left eye and is Type I diabetic?

12. What are the codes for a patient who has epilepsy marked by grand mal seizures which is not responding to treatment?

13. What are the codes for a patient who has tic douloureux?

14. What are the codes for a patient who has pseudocyesis?

15. What are the codes for a patient who has Huntington's dementia?

TEST 1

1.   What are the codes for a patient with senile dementia?

2.   What are the codes for a patient who has sickle cell anemia Hb-SS with acute chest syndrome?

3.   What is hemolysis?

4.   What are the codes for a patient who is diagnosed with anemia due to a chronic gastric ulcer?

5.   What are the codes for a patient with benign CKD stage 4 and ASCVD due to hypertension?

6.   What are the codes for a pregnant woman who has had three previous miscarriages at approximately 18 weeks and presents today at 20 weeks gestation who is experiencing cramping?

7.   What are the codes for a patient with Crohn's disease?

8.   What is the term for painful menstruation?

9.   What are the codes for a patient with oophoritis and salpingitis?

10.   What are the codes for a patient with cellulitis with possible sepsis and COPD with diabetes?

11.   What are the codes for a 2-month-old baby who presents with a diaper rash?

12.   What is the code for a patient with gastritis after ingesting Percodan with alcohol and OTC antihistamines?

13.   What is the code for a patient with scar tissue due to a second and third degree burn on both legs six months ago?

14.   What are the codes for an anemic patient due to hemorrhaging of a lower leg wound caused by a car accident?

15.   What are the codes for a patient with a stage 2 ulcer of the ankle that developed from a cast that was applied to their left lower tibia for 3 months due to a transverse fracture of the shaft?

16.   What are the codes for a patient who has pyogenic arthritis of the hip due to staph?

17.   What are the codes for a patient with acute and chronic pericarditis?

18.   What are the codes for a patient with amebic carditis?

19.   What are the codes for a patient who has right heart failure?

20.   What are dilated, swollen, painful veins in the anus or rectum known as?

21.   What are the codes for a patient with COPD and emphysema?

22.   What are the codes for a Type II diabetic patient with neuropathy and pneumonia due to MRSA and a fever?

23.   What are the codes for a patient with asthma that was precipitated by exercise?

24.   What are the codes for a patient with a perforated appendix with an abscess?

25.   What are the codes for a patient with RAD?

26.   What three things must occur for a woman to be diagnosed as having preeclampsia?

27.   What are the codes for a 36-year-old pregnant woman who has a C section due to fetal distress at 39 weeks?

28.   What is another term for delivery?

29.   What is considered a high blood pressure?

30.   What are the codes for a patient who has mitral valve stenosis with aortic valve insufficiency?

31.   What are the codes for a patient who was diagnosed nine weeks ago with chronic coronary insufficiency?

32.   What are the codes for a 25-year-old pregnant woman who is 33-weeks gestation, has gestational diabetes and is seen today for dehydration?

33.   What are the codes for an 18-year-old pregnant woman who has difficulty in labor due to the birth of a 12 pound baby boy?

34.   What are the codes for a pregnant woman who delivered liveborn twins with one normal and the other breech at 32 weeks with both weighing 5 pounds?

35.   What are the codes for a patient with ASHD and chest pain due to an MI that was treated 10 weeks ago?

36.   What are the codes for a patient with second degree sunburn?

37.   What are the codes for a patient with pilonidal cyst with abscess?

38.   What are the codes for a patient experiencing septic shock due to UTI?

39.   What are the codes for a patient with goat's milk anemia?

40.   What are the codes for a patient who metastatic cancer of the uterus?

41.   What are the codes for a patient who has nonunion fracture of the left humerus?

42.   What are the codes for a patient who has degenerative joint disease of the knee?

43.   What are the codes for a patient who is seen today for a high fever and chest congestion due to the common cold?

44.   What are the codes for a patient who has right heart failure?

45.   What are the codes for a patient who is diagnosed with pneumothorax due to gunshot wound?

46.   What are the codes for a patient who has old bucket tear of the lateral meniscus?

47.   What are the codes for a newborn who was born with a hemangioma of the neck?

48.   What are the codes when a 1750 gm baby at 28 weeks gestation is delivered due to hypertonic labor?

49.   What are the codes for a neonate who is diagnosed with diabetes?

50.   What are the codes for a baby born at 43 weeks who experienced asphyxia due to the cord wrapped around her neck?

51.   What is the code for the newborn when her mother dies during childbirth?

52.   What are the codes for a patient with second and third degree burns covering 25% of her body with 10% being third degree with infection?

53.   What causes essential hypertension?

54.   What is reactive airway disease?

55.   What are the codes for a patient with lower respiratory infection?

56.   What are the codes for an asthmatic patient with status asthmaticus and COPD?

57.   What is the code for a patient with dislocation of an artificial hip joint?

58.   What is the code for a patient with CMV infection due to transplanted liver?

59.   What is the code for a patient with anoxic brain damage resulting from their bypass graft surgery for an MI?

60.   What is the code for a patient with failure of the battery of the pacemaker after two years requiring replacement?

CHAPTER 12
ICD-10 EYE

You will learn the following in this chapter:

- A. Injuries
- J. Inflammation
- K. Foreign Body
- L. Cataracts
- M. Glaucoma
- N. Other Disorders
- O. Visual
- P. Procedural Complications

Chapter 7 is described as "Diseases of the Eye and Adnexa" and range from H00-H59. These codes have been expanded greatly with fourth, fifth and sixth characters that further describe the site and laterality. If the cause of the eye condition is known then it should be coded with the external codes.

Section 12.1: INJURIES

Many eye conditions are excluded due to other conditions as indicated by the exclude notes. Superficial injury and open wounds of the eye are coded with S00-S01 codes.

Section 12.2: INFLAMMATION

Various inflammations of the eyes are coded with H01 codes including blepharitis (ulcerative or squamous), dermatoses/dermatitis, and xeroderma which are also differentiated by laterality and upper or lower eyelid.

Conjunctivitis (H10) includes conjunctivitis that is mucopurulent, actute, atopic, toxic, serous, chronic, simple, follicular and vernal. Conjunctivitis can also include the eyelid which is known as blepharoconjunctivitis.

Iridocyclitis (H20) due to disease are not coded in this section as described in the exclude notes. Various types of iridocyclitis include primary, recurrent, hypopyon, chronic lens-induced, and other syndromes.

Section 12.3: FOREIGN BODY

Retained foreign body in the eyelid is coded as H02.81 with the use of Z codes to indicate the type of foreign body. Also contained in the H02.8 codes are cysts, dermatochalasis, edema, elephantiasis, hypertrichosis and vascular anomalies. Foreign body in the orbit is coded as H05.5. Foreign bodies in these sites (H44.6) are differentiated by if the foreign body was magnetic or not or unspecified.

Section 12.4: CATARACTS

Disorders of the lens (H25-H28) include cataracts which are now described as age-related cataract instead of senile. Cataracts are the clouding or opacification of the lens of the eye or its capsule and can result in loss of vision. Senile cataracts occur in old age when there are characteristics of impaired memory or the inability to perform certain mental tasks. Presenile cataracts occur before the period of senility which is typically 65 years of age.

Fourth characters classify conditions by type of cataract. All other types of cataracts are coded as H26 such as infantile/juvenile, traumatic, complicated, and flecks. H28 codes are for cataracts that are due to another condition.

Section 12.5: GLAUCOMA

Glaucoma contains a group of diseases of the optic nerve which is characterized by intraocular pressure and resulting in visual impairment. Glaucoma (H40) is differentiated as suspect, open-angle, primary angle-closure, secondary to trauma or inflammation, or drugs. There are boxes for seventh characters in this section for stages. Open angle occurs from an increase in the fluid pressure in the eye due to a blockage of the ocular fluid. This type of glaucoma is also described as chronic and develops slowly. Closed angle is described as acute with rapid onset due to blockage of the chamber angle where the iris and cornea meet and, therefore, the aqueous fluid cannot drain.

Section 12.6: OTHER DISORDERS

Styes (hordeolums) are coded as H00 on either the external or internal portion of the upper or lower eyelid on either the right or left side. Abscess of the eyelid and chalazion are also coded in this section.

Other disorders of the eyelid are coded as H02 such as entropion, trichiasis, ectropion, lagophthalmos, blepharochalasis, ptosis (drooping), innervation syndrome, retraction, xanethelasma, cholasma, madarosis and vitiligo.

Disorders of the lacrimal system (H04) include dacryoadenitis either acute or chronic, dacryops, dry eye syndrome, cysts, atrophy, dislocation, epiphora, inflammation, stenosis, insufficiency of lacrimal passages, fistula, and granuloma.

Disorders of the eye orbit (H05) include inflammation, displacement, edema, hemorrhage, exophthalmos, deformity due to many conditions such as disease, trauma or surgery, atrophy, enlargement, exostosis, and enophthalmos.

Other conditions of the conjunctiva (H11) includes a benign growth on it known as pterygium with specification as to exact location. Also included are codes for degeneration, deposits, concretions, xerosis, pigmentation, scars, granuloma, hemorrhage, vascular abnormalities, edema, hyperemia, cysts and conjunctivochalasis

Disorders of the sclera (H15) include scleritis and staphyloma. Disorders of the sclera (H16) include many types of keratitis, ulcers, keratoconjunctivitis, and neovascularization. Corneal scars and opacities are coded as H17.

Other disorders of the cornea (H18) include pigmentations, deposits, keratopathy, edema, changes of the membranes, degeneration, keratomalacia, arcus senilis, hereditary dystrophies, keratoconus, ectasia, staphyloma, anesthesia, hypoesthesia, disorders due to contact lens, and erosion.

Other disorders of the iris and ciliary body (H21) include hyphema, degeneration, iridoschisis, cysts, pupillary membranes, adhesions, and floppy iris syndrome.

Other disorders of the lens (H27) include aphakia which is absence of the lens and dislocation.

Disorders of the choroid and retina (H30-H36) include inflammation, cyclitis, Harada's disease, scars, retinopathy, degeneration, atrophy, hemorrhage, rupture, cysts, retinoschisis, occlusions, changes in appearance, aneurysms, vasculitis, hemorrhages, separation, and detachment. Retinal detachment is coded as H33 which include single or multiple breaks. Retinopathy in premature babies is coded as H35.1 and is differentiated by stages. Proliferative retinopathy not due to diabetes is coded as H35.2. Macular degeneration, (loss of central vision) is coded as H35.3. Peripheral retinal degeneration is coded as H35.4. H40 is highly specific for glaucoma differentiated by stages, tension, and laterality.

Disorders of the vitreous body and globe (H43-H44) include prolapse, hemorrhage, crystalline deposits, opacities, adhesions, degeneration, endophthalmitis, and hypotony.

Disorders of the optic nerve and visual pathways (H46-H47) include neuritis, neuropathy, hypoplasia, hemorrhage, papilledema, atrophy, coloboma, inflammation, cortical blindness, or due to neoplasm.

Other disorders of the eyes (H55-H57) include nystagmus, anomalies such as mydriasis, and pain.

Section 12.7: VISUAL

Disorders of ocular muscles, binocular movement, accommodation and refraction (H49-H52) include strabismus. Strabismus is the inability of the both eyes to look in the same direction due to muscle weakness of one eye. Strabismus is coded as paralytic, esotropia either alternating or monocular, exotropia, vertical, intermittent heterotropia heterophoria, and mechanical.

Other disorders include binocular movement, refraction, accommodation, myopia (nearsightedness), astigmatism (defective curvature of the cornea or lens), hyperopia (farsightedness), and presbyopia (impairment of vision due to old age).

Visual disturbances (H53-H54) include amblyopia, discomfort, sudden visual loss, transient vision loss, day blindness, diplopia, scotoma, defects, contraction of visual field, color vision deficiencies, and night blindness.

Also coded in this section is blindness and low vision (H54) with fourth characters classifying which eyes are involved and if there is blindness or low vision, e.g. blindness in both eyes are coded as H54.0 and blindness in one eye and low vision in the other is coded as H54.1. If a cause is known for the blindness, the code instructs the additional coding of the underlying cause. Legal blindness is coded as H54.8. Visual impairment is differentiated as 1, 2, 3, 4, 5 or 9 depending on visual acuity with 5 indicating no light perception and 9 undetermined or unspecified.

Section 12.8: PROCEDURAL COMPLICATIONS

Complications and disorders to the eyes due to a procedure either during the procedure or after are coded as H59 which include keratopathy, fragments in the eyes, edema, hemorrhage, hematoma, accidental puncture or laceration, inflammation, and scars.

CHAPTER 13
ICD-10 EAR

You will learn the following in this chapter:

B. Otitis
  1. Suppurative
  2. Serous
  3. Otitis Media
  4. Otitis Externa
Q. Diseases
  5. Inner Ear
  6. External Ear
  7. Middle Ear
R. Other Disorders
S. Procedural Complications

Chapter 8 is described as "Diseases of the Ear and Mastoid Process" and range from H60-H95. These codes are broken into five blocks: external ear, middle ear and mastoid, inner ear, other disorders, and intraoperative and postprocedural complications.

Section 13.1: OTITIS

There are various disorders of the ear which include tinnitus (ringing sensation in the ears), vertigo, deafness, and otitis media. Otitis media is inflammation of the ear. There are two types of otitis media: suppurative is characterized by the accumulation of pus due to an infection and serous is characterized by an accumulation of serous fluid. It is important that otitis media is treated immediately as it can result in hearing impairment or loss. There is also otitis externa which is inflammation of the outer ear and is also known as swimmer's ear. Diseases of the middle ear are coded as H65-H75 such as suppurative otitis media (H66.0) and chronic serous otitis media (H65.2).

There is much greater specificity as to site and laterality through the use of fourth, fifth, and sixth characters for these codes, acute and subacute allergic otitis media (mucoid) (sanguinous) (serous), right ear (H65.111). There are also many more "code first underlying disease" notes.

Section 13.2: DISEASES

Diseases of the inner ear are coded as H80-H83. Other disorders are coded as H90-H94.

Diseases of the external ear (H60-H62) include otitis externa which can involve abscesses, cellulitis, hemorrhagic, swimmer's ear, cholesteatoma, noninfective (from chemicals, actinic, contact, eczematoid, etc), chronditis, hematomas, acquired deformities, impacted cerumen, stenosis and due to other diseases.

Diseases of the middle ear and mastoid (H65-H75) include nonsuppurative otitis media (serous and mucoid), suppurative (producing pus), in diseases classified elsewhere, salpingitis or obstruction in Eustachian tube, myringitis, atrophic flaccid or nonflaccid tympanic membrane, sclerosis, adhesive disease, discontinuity, dislocation, ankylosis or loss of ear ossicles, polyp, mastoiditis, and cholesteatoma. If the tympanic membrane has been perforated, code H72 should be used in addition to instructions to code first any associated otitis media.

Diseases of the inner ear (H80-H83) include otosclerosis, Meniere's Disease, vertigo, neuronitis, other diseases of the inner ear, and noise effect conditions.

Section 13.3: OTHER DISORDERS

Other disorders of the ear (H90-H94) include hearing losses (conductive, sensorineural, mixed, ototoxic, and presbycusis) otalgia, effusion (otorrhea), otorrhagia, degeneration, deafness, tinnitus, hyperacusis, in other diseases, and temporary loss of hearing.

Section 13.4: PROCEDURAL COMPLICATIONS

Codes for intraoperative or postprocedural complications are coded as H95.

CHAPTER 14
ICD-10 CIRCULATORY SYSTEM

You will learn the following objectives in this chapter:

A. Circulatory System
B. Rheumatic Fever/Heart Disease
C. Hypertension
D. Ischemic Heart Disease
E. Diseases of Pulmonary Circulation
F. Other Forms of Heart Disease
    1. Pericarditis/Endocarditis/Myocarditis
    2. Conduction Disorders
    3. Dysrhythmias
    4. Heart Failure
    5. Cerebrovascular Diseases
G. Diseases of the Arteries
H. Diseases of the Veins
I.   Other
J. Operative Complications

CIRCULATORY SYSTEM: Chapter 9 is described as "Diseases of the Circulatory System" and range from I00-I99. Remember, these are I's, not the number one.

Section 14.1: CIRCULATORY SYSTEM

nih.gov

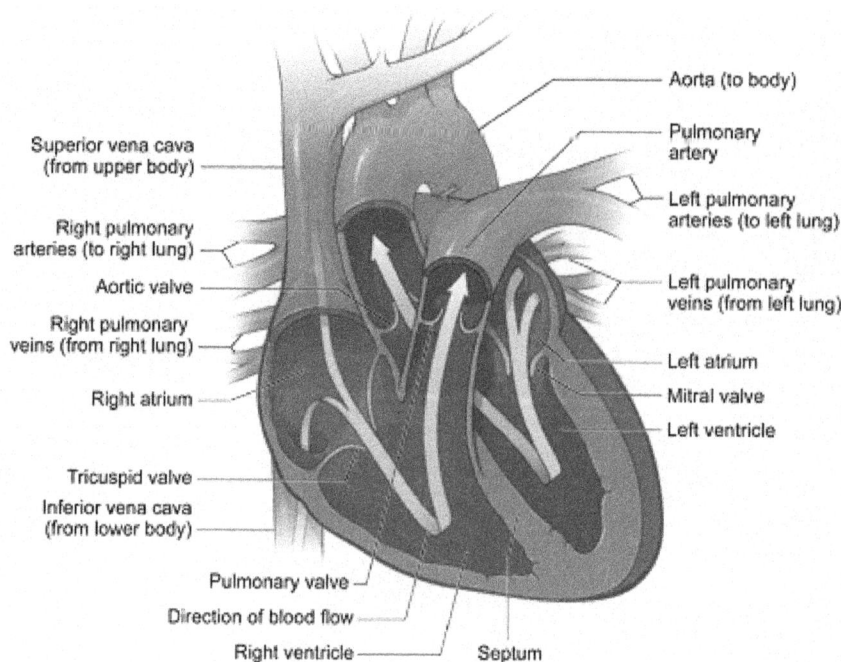

The circulatory system is extensive and so is the complexity of the coding that accompanies it. In fact, some of the most proficient coders are cardiovascular coders. This complexity is due to the vast vascular system of which knowing the anatomy and physiology is a great challenge, in addition to multitude, severity, and prominence of related diseases and conditions and the complexity and rapid advancements in procedures.

The cardiovascular system is comprised of the heart and the vascular system. The cardiovascular system is the means by which all nutrients, water, and oxygen are distributed to the rest of our body.

The vascular system is comprised of a hierarchial system of blood vessels. Arteries are the larger blood vessels that carry oxygen-rich blood away from the heart and is the color red. Once the blood has been depleted of oxygen, nutrients, and water, the blood returns to the heart through the veins.

It is important to understand the flow of the blood, not only through the arteries and veins, but also through the heart and will continue to be very critical in the selection of CPT codes. Blood flow begins when the blood enters the right atrium of the heart:

(1) Blood enters the right atrium (upper) of the heart through the superior vena cava from the upper portions of the body and through the inferior vena cava from the lower portions of the body.
(2) Blood then passes through the tricuspid valve into the right ventricle of the heart.
(3) Blood then passes through the pulmonary valve into the pulmonary artery and into the lungs where it is enriched with oxygen. This is the only artery of the body that contains oxygen-poor blood which is blue.
(4) The blood then returns from the lungs now rich with oxygen through the pulmonary vein and into the left atrium. This is the only vein of the body that contains oxygen-rich blood and is red.
(5) The blood then passes through the mitral valve into the left ventricle.
(6) The blood then passes out of the left ventricle through the aortic valve and into the aorta, then into the rest of the body through the arterial system.

LAYERS OF HEART: There are three layers to the heart, the endocardium which lines the interior of the heart, the myocardium which is the thick muscular middle portion of the heart, and the pericardium which surrounds the heart.

PHASES: There are two phases to a heartbeat: diastole and systole. Diastole is the phase when the ventricles are relaxing and the heart is filling with blood. Systole is when the ventricles are contracting and pushing blood into the pulmonary artery and aorta. The phases are indicated by the blood pressure reading in which the systole number is on top and the diastole number is on the bottom as a fraction. For example, blood pressure of 120/80 means the systole is 120 and the diastole is 80. Blood pressure in which the systole rate is sustained at above 140 and/or a diastole rate is sustained above 90 is considered hypertension and constitutes a health risk. An abnormal heart rate is known as a murmur.

CONDUCTION: The heartbeat is initiated by an electrical impulse from the sinoatrial node (SA node) located in the right atrium. It is also known as pacemaker, albeit the natural one and not an implanted pacemaker. This electrical impulse causes the atrium to contract and push blood into the ventricle; thereby, starting the flow of the blood through the heart and the continuing ripple of the electricity throughout the heart. This electrical impulse then passes to the atrioventricular node (AV node), to the AV bundle (bundle of His), which then divides into the right and left bundle branches. These terms are important when coding as blockages of these areas can result in serious health issues.

Section 14.2: RHEUMATIC FEVER/HEART DISEASE

Rheumatic fever is a sequela of a streptococcal infection, group A, and can result in serious damage to the heart, known as rheumatic heart disease. It occurs most often in younger people.

Rheumatic fever can be coded alone if it the heart is not involved, as described by the physician. The codes are also distinguished by which layer of the heart is involved: pericarditis is inflammation of the outer layer; endocarditis is inflammation of the inner layer; and myocarditis which is inflammation of the middle layer.

These conditions can be acute or chronic. The physician must describe it as chronic to be listed as chronic; otherwise, it would be coded as acute which means the condition is currently occurring.

The inflammation from the infection and fever can result in damage to the valves, including stenosis, which can be heard as a murmur during a cardiac examination. Most oftentimes it is the mitral valve that is damaged. The codes are distinguished by which valve is damaged.

Acute rheumatic heart disease or rheumatic chorea are coded as I00-I09 and are further specified as to with or without heart involvement. Chronic rheumatic heart disease is coded as I05-I09. Other rheumatic heart disease include myocarditis, pericarditis and heart failure. There are notes indicating the need to code additional codes for type of condition such as heart failure.

Rheumatic valvular disease is coded as I05-I09 for the mitral valve, arotic valve, and tricuspid which can involve multiple valves together. Rheumatic valvular disease can include stenosis or insufficiency. ICD-10 assumes that valvular disease was caused by rheumatic heart fever caused by streptococci unless it is described as non-rheumatic (I34). Only aortic valvular disease is assumed to be non-rheumatic unless otherwise stated.

Section 14.3: HYPERTENSION

Hypertension is the elevation of the blood pressure, either or both the systole and diastole pressures. Hypertension is considered a major factor in atherosclerosis, cardiovascular disease, heart failure, coronary artery disease, and stroke. Hypertension is certainly a condition that complicates the care of the patient, so if a patient is described as having hypertension by the physician, then it is usually coded even if the hypertension is not the main reason for the visit nor does the patient receive any care for it.

Hypertension is coded as I10-I15. It is specified as it was previously in ICD-9, i.e. primary or secondary and with or without heart or renal involvement. However, there is no specification of type of hypertension (malignant, benign, or unspecified). Fourth characters further classify the hypertension codes as to presence of congestive heart failure and renal failure. When a patient has only high blood pressure with no diagnosis of hypertension (also known as transient hypertension) it is coded as R03.0.

The great majority of hypertension is primary (essential) and its cause is not known. The remainder is secondary to renal disease which is due to the physiological relatedness of the renal system and blood pressure. The condition causing the hypertension should also be coded (multiple coding).

There is no longer a table in the alphabetical index for hypertension.

Additional codes should be listed for exposure to tobacco smoke.

There are separate codes for a hypertensive condition in a pregnant mother (O10-O11) which is known as transient. A hypertensive condition in the baby is coded as P92.2. This is an important distinction because a mother may develop hypertension while pregnant but it is only transient due to the pregnancy and should cease once she is no longer pregnant.

There are several scenarios for coding hypertension codes when heart or kidney conditions are occurring at the same time. First, the term hypertension may be described as a diagnosis in addition to a heart condition, but they are not described as related. If the physician does not link these two conditions with statements such as "hypertensive heart disease" or "heart disease complicated by hypertension", etc, then you must code the heart condition and the hypertension separately. However, if the physician does describe the hypertension and heart condition as being related, such as "hypertensive heart disease" or "due to", then I11 should be used. The code directs the additional coding of the heart problem. Hypertension can affect the heart because it causes the heart to work harder which results in thickening of the left ventricle and can result in heart failure.

WARNING: The use of conjunctions may be confusing so beware! If a physician describes a condition as "heart problem with hypertension," the "with" may not necessarily mean that the two conditions are related to each other although the hypertension codes do use the "with" to denote a relationship. Therefore, you should check with a physician or check the report for further information to be sure if the heart condition and hypertension should be coded with one code if they are related.

The term hypertension may be described as a diagnosis in addition to a renal (kidney) condition. If the renal condition is described as acute and the physician does not describe the renal condition being related to the hypertension, then the two conditions are coded separately (as we did with the heart condition).

However, if the renal condition is chronic, then hypertension and the renal condition are coded as related. Chronic renal conditions are considered related to hypertension because the hypertension causes damage to the kidneys. This is also known as hypertensive nephropathy, hypertensive nephrosclerosis, hypertensive renal disease, chronic renal disease (CRD), or chronic kidney disease (CKD). If the renal condition is chronic, then the hypertension and renal disease are related and code them together in one code (I13) even if the doctor does not define them as being related, such as if he said hypertension and chronic renal disease. In addition, another code is needed for the renal disease and its stage as denoted in the hypertension notes in the coding book. Renal diseases codes are differentiated by stages with stage V being end stage renal disease (ESRD).

A physician may describe both a heart and renal condition as being related to hypertension, and this is also coded with I13 codes. This is also known as cardiorenal hypertension.

Secondary hypertension is coded as I15.

Section 14.4: ISCHEMIC HEART DISEASE

Ischemic heart disease is caused by arteriosclerotic heart disease (ASHD) (I70) in that the arteries of the heart are hardened and narrowed, resulting in coronary ischemia and coronary artery disease (CAD). This occurs when atherosclerosis causes a lack of blood flow (ischemia) and, therefore, a lack of oxygen which can result in impaired functions, infarctions, or necrosis (death). The area of dead tissue is known as an infarction (not infraction). Chest pain is known as angina pectoris.

Heart problems may be indicated by Mobitz II heart block, ventricular fibrillation and angina pectoris (chest pain, I20) which can be unstable or with spasms.

If this infarction is of the heart, it is known as a myocardial infarction (MI) and is also known as a heart attack or cardiac arrest. MIs are coded with I22 codes if the duration is less than four weeks. The codes are based on where the ST elevation (STEMI) is in the heart or if there is non-ST elevation (NSTEMI). Additional codes are also required for tobacco exposure and if status post administration of tPA within last 24 hours at another facility.

Cardiac arrest (I46) occurs when the heart stops. Heart attack refers to a blockage in a coronary artery resulting in heart muscle damage and is commonly known as a myocardial infarction (MI) (I21). It is important to understand the differences between heart attack, cardiac arrest, and heart failure.

If a subsequent MI occurs within four weeks after a previous MI, then the correct codes would be I22. Certain complications to the MI should be coded additionally with I23 codes such as atrial septal defect, rupture of cardiac wall, and thrombosis of atrium.

If ischemic heart disease does not result in an MI, then codes I24 should be used, such as a thrombosis or postmyocardial infarction syndrome.

If the patient is diagnosed as having an old or healed MI or if an MI was diagnosed on an EKG (ECG) but is not presenting any problems at this time, it should be coded with I25.2.

Chronic ischemic heart disease (I25) includes atherosclerosis. Atherosclerosis precedes arteriosclerosis in that atherosclerosis is the accumulation of fatty deposits in the arterial system. This then results in arteriosclerosis, which is hardening of the arteries due to the development of plaque from the fatty deposits. With these deposits of plaque, a clot can form which is known as a thrombosis. If this thrombosis dislodges and is released into the rest of the arterial system it is known as an embolus and can be deadly.

Within the codes, atherosclerosis can be defined with angina pectoris or spasms and occurring in a native artery or area with a bypass graft or of a transplanted heart. Chronic total occlusion of a coronary artery is coded as I25.82 which can be coded in addition to atherosclerosis.

Aneurysms (I25.3) are weakened areas of the vascular walls which can result in rupture. NOTE that although hyperlipidemia (elevation of fats in the blood) and hypercholesterolemia (high levels of cholesterol in the blood) are major factors in the development of arteriosclerosis and hypertension, they are coded from endocrine/metabolic codes.

Section 14.5: DISEASES OF PULMONARY CIRCULATION

Diseases of the pulmonary circulation (I26-I28) refer to conditions related to the pulmonary vein or artery, such as arteriosclerosis, hypertension, aneurysm, infarction, and embolism. Remember that iatrogenic means the condition resulted from medical care.

Pulmonary embolisms are coded as I26 if it not related to surgery or is a complication of pregnancy.

There are references in some descriptions of the codes to septic involvement which needs to also be coded, as described in an earlier packet and as noted in the ICD-10 book.

An arteriovenous fistula (I28.0) is an abnormal connection or passageway between an artery and a vein. Aneurysm of the pulmonary artery is coded as I28.1.

Section 14.6: PERICARDITIS/ENDOCARDITIS/MYOCARDITIS

Pericarditis (I30) is inflammation of the sac surrounding the heart; endocarditis (I33) is inflammation of the interior tissue of the heart; and myocarditis (I40) is inflammation of the heart muscle. Inflammation can be due to an infectious organism or idiopathic which means the cause is unknown. Remember, you must code the organism also, if known. Many of these codes include acute and subacute. Subacute refers to a condition being less severe or having less duration than an acute condition and not long enough to be considered chronic.

Disorders of valves include insufficiency, incompetence, regurgitation, and endocarditis of the mitral valve (I34), the aortic valve (I35), the tricuspid valve (I36), and the pulmonary valve (I37). Incompetence can result from stenosis, which is narrowing of the valves and the failure of the valve to operate properly. Insufficiency and regurgitation occurs when the valve allows backward flow of blood.

Cardiomyopathy is disease involving the heart (I42). Cardiomyopathy may be due to many factors, such as diseases, arteriosclerosis, alcohol abuse, nutritional deficiencies, and diseases.

Section 14.7: CONDUCTION DISORDERS

Conduction codes (I44) include such terms as left bundle branch block and atrioventricular (AV) blocks. The bundle of His branches into three bundle branches, the right, left anterior and left posterior bundle branches which can experience blockage causing a defect in the electrical system of the heart. RBBB is a right bundle branch block and LBBB is a left bundle branch block. AV blocks involve impairment of the conduction from the atrium to the ventricular Bundle of His. There are three types of AV blocks: in the first degree AV block there is a slowing of the conduction as noted on an EKG as a prolonged PR interval; a second degree AV block, also known as Mobitz I or II, or Wenckebach, involves a greater slowing of the conduction and some missed beats; third degree AV block, also known as a complete heart block, occurs when there is complete blockage of the conduction from the atria to the ventricle. Usually this requires the implantation of a pacemaker.

Peripheral vascular disease (PVD) is included in this section (I44). PVD is any disease caused by obstruction of the arteries in the legs and arms. It is also known as peripheral artery disease (PAD) or peripheral artery occlusive disease (PAOD).

Section 14.8: DYSRHYTHMIAS

Cardiac dysrhythmias (I48-I49) are abnormal electrical currents in the heart which can result in irregular, slowed, or fast heart beats. These codes are differentiated by being supraventricular or ventricular. Supraventricular are those arrhythmias generated within the SA node, atria, and AV node. Ventricular are those arrhythmias generated in the ventricular conduction system. The result of dysrhythmias can include tachycardia (fast heartbeat), bradycardia (slow heart beat), and fibrillation/flutter (disorganized current flow).

Section 14.9: HEART FAILURE

Heart failure (I50) is the insufficiency of the heart to pump adequate amounts of blood. Differentiation of codes is based on congestive heart failure which includes right heart failure due to left heart failure since heart failure usually begins in the left heart and then progresses to the right. Because the failure can begin in the left, there is a code for left heart failure only (I50.1). The codes are also differentiated based on systolic or diastolic heart failure. There are many notes about coding first for a variety of reasons including following surgery or hypertension.

Section 14.10: CEREBROVASCULAR DISEASES

Cerebrovascular diseases (I60-I69) refer to conditions pertaining to the blood vessels or blood flow to the brain through the vascular system. These include hemorrhages (bleeding), occlusion (closure due to blockage), stenosis (narrowing), and ischemia (restriction in blood flow). These codes are usually referenced by the artery involved.

There are many additional codes that need to be coded if present which includes alcohol abuse, exposure to tobacco, and hypertension.

Nontraumatic subarachnoid hemorrhages are further specified by site, e.g. nontraumatic subarachnoid hemorrhage from carotid siphon and bifurcation, I60.0.

Embolism and thrombus are listed under occlusion because they cause an occlusion, thus resulting in a cerebral infarction (I63). These occlusions, stenosis, or hemorrhaging (known as aneurysms) can result in a cerebrovascular accident (CVA), better known as a stroke. CVA is a lack of blood to the brain which can result in the loss of brain functions and related activities, such as speech, motor ability and vision.

Transient cerebral ischemia (TIA) (G45.9) is a temporary loss of blood to the brain, as transient means temporary, and is not coded from this section.

Stroke is coded as I63.9. Sequelae from a CVA are coded as I69 plus a code for the specific condition. Late effects of cerebrovascular diseases (I69) have been expanded to include laterality, trauma, site, dominance, and deficits, e.g. monoplegia of upper limb following nontraumatic subarachnoid hemorrhage affecting right dominant side, I69.031. A late effect is a sequela or residual that is caused by an acute condition but which remains after the treatment of the acute condition is completed.

Section 14.11: DISEASES OF THE ARTERIES

These codes (I70-I79) include conditions involving the arteries, arterioles and capillaries, such as atherosclerosis, aneurysm, embolism, thrombus, polyarteritis, and fistulas.

These codes are further classified by additional complications, such as claudication (cramps in the legs caused by poor circulation within the arteries), rest pain, ulceration, and gangrene.

Section 14.12: DISEASES OF VEINS AND OTHERS

These codes, I80-I89, include some of the conditions previously described in the arterial system, such as embolism for veins, lymphatic vessels, and lymph nodes, but does contain other categories.

Phlebitis and thrombophlebitis (I80.0) are inflammation of veins and creation of thrombus and are classified by the veins involved.

Varicose veins (I83) of the lower extremities are veins that have become enlarged and tortuous because the valves that prevent the backward flow of blood no longer functioning properly and so a leakage of blood occurs. Not only can this cause unsightly veins which become enlarged, but it can result in ulceration which is a disruption in the layers of the skin so that a sore appears. The codes are differentiated by the presence of ulcers, inflammation or other complications. There are separate codes for varicose veins of other anatomic sites, such as gastric (I86.4) which can be deadly.

Hemorrhoids (K64) are contained in the digestive system chapter. They are dilated, swollen, painful veins in the anus or rectum. These can be complicated by thrombosis, bleeding, strangulation, ulceration, and prolapse (falling down or slipping out of place). They are classified as internal or external. External hemorrhoids protrude from the rectum through the anus.

Section 14.13: OTHER

Lymphadenitis (I88) has been moved to this section of codes. Gangrene has also been moved to this section (I96). Hypotension (I95.9) is an abnormally low blood pressure which can be caused by various conditions such as hemodialysis, drugs, idiopathic (origin not known) or postprocedural.

Section 14.14: OPERATIVE COMPLICATIONS

Intraoperative and postprocedural complications are coded as I97 and include hemorrhage, hematoma, puncture, laceration, cardiac insufficiency, cardiac arrest, heart failure, and cerebrovascular infarction.

CIRCULATORY QUIZ 8

1. What are the codes for a patient with congestive heart failure and hypertension?

2. What are the codes for a patient with elevated blood pressure?

3. What are the codes for a patient with malignant hypertensive stage IV CKD?

4. What are the codes for a patient with benign CKD stage 4 and ASCVD due to hypertension?

5. What are the codes for a patient with acute and chronic pericarditis?

6. What are the codes for a patient who has a complete AV heart block?

7. What are the codes for a patient who has strangulated internal hemorrhoids with bleeding?

8. What are the codes for a patient who has hemiplegia after experiencing a CVA 6 months ago?

9. What are the codes for a patient who was diagnosed nine weeks ago with chronic coronary insufficiency?

10. What are the codes for a patient who had an appendectomy due to appendicitis who has postoperative hypertension?

11. What are the codes for a patient who is not presenting with any symptoms but was diagnosed as having MI on an EKG reading?

12. What are the codes for a patient diagnosed with intermediate coronary syndrome?

13. What are the codes for a patient with chest pain due to acute MI of the inferoposterior wall as part of initial care?

14. What are the codes for a patient with RBBB?

15. What are the codes for a patient who has aplastic anemia due to radiation therapy?

CHAPTER 15
ICD-10 RESPIRATORY SYSTEM

You will learn the following objectives in this chapter:

A. Respiratory System
B. Acute Respiratory Infections
C. Upper Respiratory Tract Conditions
D. Pneumonia/Influenza
E. Acute Lower Respiratory Infections
F. Other Upper Respiratory Infections
G. Chronic Lower Respiratory Infections
H. Chronic Obstructive Pulmonary Disease
I. Other Lung Diseases Due to External Agents
J. Other Respiratory Diseases
K. Suppurative and Necrotic Conditions
L. Procedural Complications

Chapter 10 is described as "Diseases of the Respiratory System" and range from J00-J99.

Section 15.1: RESPIRATORY SYSTEM
The respiratory system includes airways, lungs, and the respiratory muscles and the process of allowing gas exchange (respiration), primarily of oxygen and carbon dioxide. Respiration consists of internal and external respiration. External respiration involves the lungs and the air sacs of the lung. Internal respiration involves the exchange of gases at the cellular level in which oxygen passes into the cells and carbon dioxide passes out so that it can be exhaled from the body through the lungs.

Air enters through the nose and proceeds through the pharynx (throat). The nose area contains the sinuses, which include the maxillary, frontal, ethmoidal, and sphenoidal. The pharynx is comprised of the nasopharynx where the tonsils and adenoids are located, then into the oropharynx, and lastly the laryngopharynx. The laryngopharynx divides into two branches, the larynx (voice box) and the esophagus. While the esophagus leads into the stomach, the larynx leads into the lungs. The epiglottis is a flap that controls the opening of the laryngopharynx so that either the larynx or the esophagus branch is open.

PARANASAL SINUSES: The paranasal sinuses are the frontal, maxillary, ethmoid and sphenoid.

Sphenoid sinus

Frontal sinus

Ethmoid sinus

Maxillary sinus

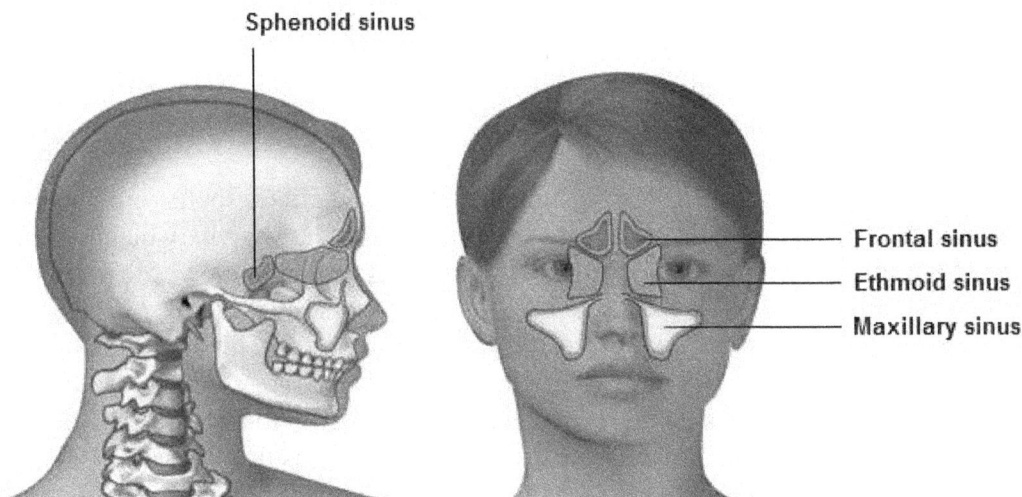

National Pain Foundation

The larynx then opens into the trachea (windpipe) which branches into the bronchial tubes (bronchi) thus leading into the right and left lungs. These then branch into bronchioles which end in clusters of air sacs called alveoli. It is here that the exchange of gases occur with the capillaries so that oxygen can pass into the blood and be dispersed to the cells. (American Lung Association)

Each lung is covered by the membranous pleura. The outer layer is called the parietal pleura and the inner layer is called the visceral pleura (surrounding an organ).

The diaphragm is a muscle that separates the thoracic cavity from the abdominal cavity. It is involved in the inhalation and exhalation of the lungs through contractions.

The right lung is divided into three lobes and the left lung has two lobes, so they are not mirror images of each other and cannot be coded as bilateral if a procedure is done on both sides.

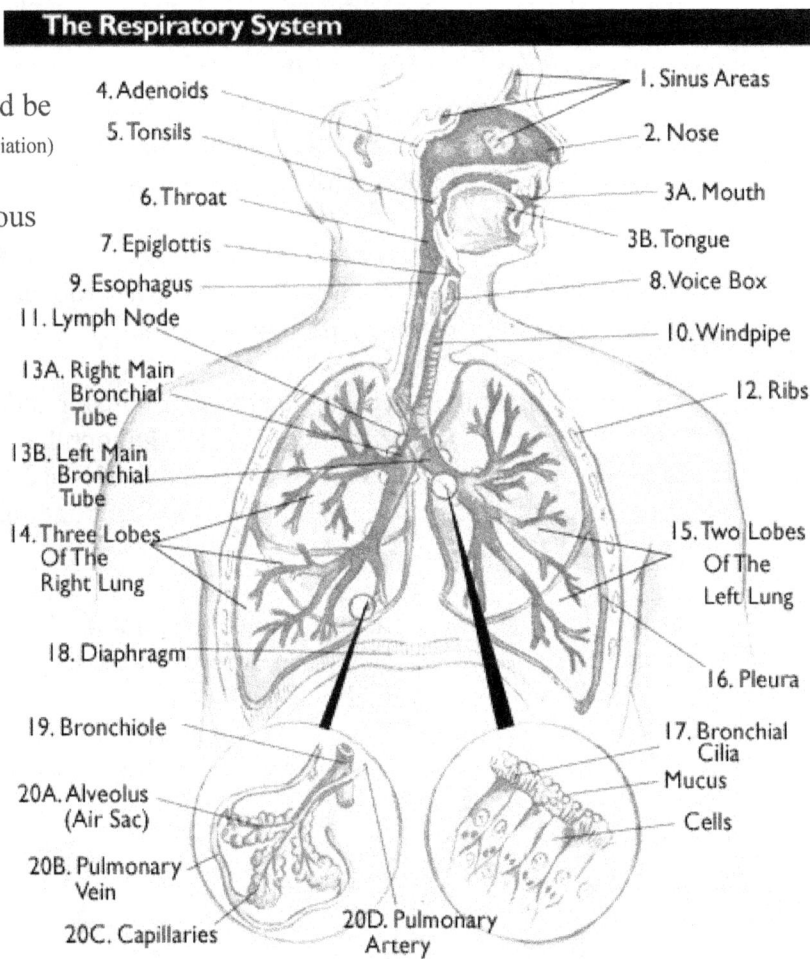

The Respiratory System

4. Adenoids
5. Tonsils
6. Throat
7. Epiglottis
9. Esophagus
11. Lymph Node
13A. Right Main Bronchial Tube
13B. Left Main Bronchial Tube
14. Three Lobes Of The Right Lung
18. Diaphragm
19. Bronchiole
20A. Alveolus (Air Sac)
20B. Pulmonary Vein
20C. Capillaries
20D. Pulmonary Artery

1. Sinus Areas
2. Nose
3A. Mouth
3B. Tongue
8. Voice Box
10. Windpipe
12. Ribs
15. Two Lobes Of The Left Lung
16. Pleura
17. Bronchial Cilia
Mucus
Cells

Section 15.2: ACUTE RESPIRATORY INFECTIONS

For all codes in this chapter, when a respiratory condition occurs in more than one site, if there is not a code specifying these multiple sites, then the lowest anatomic site location should be used to select the code as noted in the book.

Acute respiratory infections (J00-J06) include the common cold (nasopharyngitis) (J00), sinusitis (inflammation of the sinuses), pharyngitis (inflammation of the pharynx which includes sore throat), tonsillitis (inflammation of the tonsils), laryngitis (inflammation of the larynx), bronchitis (inflammation of the bronchial tubes), and bronchiolitis (inflammation of the bronchioles). Croup is coded as J05, acute obstructive laryngitis with or without obstruction.

Tonsillitis codes have been expanded to include organisms with the fourth character and the level (acuity or recurrent) with the fifth character, e.g. acute tonsillitis due to other specified organisms (J03.80). Pharyngitis similarly has been expanded in the fourth character to specify the organism, e.g. acute pharyngitis due to strep (J02.0). Remember, the organism should also be coded, in addition.

Section 15.3: UPPER RESPIRATORY TRACT CONDITIONS

Acute upper respiratory infections (URI) of multiple or unspecified sites are coded as J06. Acute (LRI) is coded as J22. Chronic lower respiratory infection is coded as chronic bronchitis.

Section 15.4: PNEUMONIA/INFLUENZA

Influenza and pneumonia are coded as J09-J18. Fourth characters provide classification based on presence of pneumonia and manifestations, such as myocarditis.

Influenza is coded according to what type of virus is involved and some manifestations such as gastrointestinal or respiratory. There are notes to code the virus for some of the codes as well as to additionally code pleural effusion or sinusitis.

Pneumonia is inflammation of the lung that produces exudates. These codes are differentiated as viral (J12), Strep (J13), other bacterial (J15), Hemophilus (J14), staph (J15.2) as well as others. Notice that pneumonia due to MRSA is coded as J15.212. Pneumonia due to other diseases classified elsewhere is coded as J17 such as Q fever and rheumatic fever with a note to code the disease first.

Other types of pneumonia include bronchopneumonia (J18.0), lobar (J18.1) and hypostatic (J18.2) (hypostasis is pooling of the blood in the area of the body closest to the ground). J69 describes pneumonitis due to solids and liquids.

Section 15.5: ACUTE LOWER RESPIRATORY INFECTIONS

Acute lower respiratory infections (J20-J22) include acute and subacute bronchitis and bronchiolitis which can be differentiated by organism.

Section 15.6: OTHER UPPER RESPIRATORY TRACT DISEASES

These codes contain many of the chronic conditions, as well as conditions such as polyps (nonmalignant growth or tumor), deviation, hypertrophy (overgrowth), abscesses (collection of pus due to the body's reaction to an infection), allergic responses, paralysis, edema (swelling), stenosis, and cellulitis.

Allergic rhinitis is coded as J30 differentiated by what the cause is, such as food, animals, or pollen. Chronic rhinitis (J31) include pharyngitis and nasopharyngitis which requires the use of additional codes for any exposure to tobacco.

Chronic sinusitis (J32) is differentiated by which part of the sinus is involved such as frontal, maxillary, ethmoidal, or sphenoidal. If all sinuses are involved, then it is coded as pansinusitis, but if only some of the sinuses are involved, this would be coded as other (J32.8).

Nasal polyps are coded as J33 and other disorders of the nose and nasal sinuses (J34) include abscess, furuncle, carbuncle, cyst or deviated nasal septum.

Chronic diseases of the tonsils and adenoids (J35) include tonsillitis, adenoiditis, and hypertrophy which can be coded singly or together. Chronic laryngitis/laryngotracheitis is coded as J37.

Disease of the vocal cords and larynx (J38) include paralysis, polyp, nodules, abscess, cellulitis, leukoplakia, edema, spasm, or stenosis.

Section 15.7: CHRONIC LOWER RESPIRATORY INFECTIONS

Chronic lower respiratory infections (J40-J47) begin with bronchitis (J40) specified as neither chronic nor acute, chronic bronchitis (J41-J42) described as simple, mucopurulent or mixed simple and emphysema (J43) (chronic respiratory condition characterized by loss of elasticity of lung tissue which results in the collapse of the airways).

Chronic obstructive pulmonary disease (COPD) codes have changed in that the term COPD is now included with the chronic condition. COPD is a general term which has been used to indicate any disorder that persistently obstructs bronchial airflow. COPD is coded as J44 which includes chronic bronchitis, emphysema, and chronic asthma. You can now code COPD in addition to other chronic pulmonary diseases as indicated in the notes; some will require that you code the other condition as well such as emphysema.

Asthma (J45) includes many types including atopic, extrinsic, and idiosyncratic and can include bronchitis and rhinitis. Asthma is a chronic respiratory condition characterized by inflammation, airflow obstruction, and bronchospasm, also known as reactive airway disease (RAD). Extrinsic asthma is caused by factors outside of the body such as food allergies, while intrinsic asthma is caused by internal factors. Asthma can also be induced by exercising or coughing.

Code J45, asthma, has a fourth character for degree of persistence such as mild, moderate or persistent and either persistent or intermittent. It also has a fifth character classification that is uncomplicated, exacerbated or with status asthmaticus which is an acute attack in which the asthma is not relieved by usual treatments. Status asthmaticus is also known as intractable, refractory, and severe prolonged. There is no longer specification in the asthma codes to specify extrinsic, intrinsic, chronic obstructive and unspecified (J45).

Bronchiectasis (J47) can be coded as with acute lower respiratory infection, exacerbated, or uncomplicated

Section 15.8: LUNG DISEASES DUE TO EXTERNAL AGENTS

Various lung diseases that can be caused by external agents (J60-J70) include coalworker's pneumoconiosis, black lung disease, anthracosis, pneumoconiosis due to asbestos, silica, inorganic dusts, or tuberculosis.

Specific codes are provided for diseases or hypersensitivity (allergy) caused by organic dust (J66-J67) such as flax-dresser's disease, farmer's lung, bird fancier's lung, maple-bark-stripper's lung, air conditioner lung, or cheese-washer's lung.

Inhalation of chemicals, gases, fumes and vapors can cause various respiratory conditions (J68) including bronchitis, pneumonitis, and URI. The cause should be coded first with T51-T65 codes. Any associated respiratory conditions should also be coded such as respiratory failure (J96).

Pneumonia can be caused by the inhalation of solids and liquids into the lungs (J69) which can include food, vomit, oils and essences.

Other external agents that can cause respiratory conditions (J70) include radiation, drugs, and smoke inhalation.

Section 15.9: OTHER RESPIRATORY DISEASES

Other respiratory diseases principally affecting the interstitium (J80-J84) include acute respiratory distress syndrome, pulmonary edema, eosinophilia, fibrosis, idiopathic pneumonia, and hyperplasia. Acute Respiratory Distress Syndrome (ARDS) is coded as J80. ARDS is a serious reaction to injuries of the lung and result in inflammation, hypoxemia and can result in multiple organ failure.Empyema is coded as J86.9 and involves infection with pus in the lungs and is not the same as emphysema. Pleurisy is inflammation of the pleura.

Section 15.10: SUPPPURATIVE AND NECROTIC CONDITIONS OF LOWER RESPIRATORY TRACT

Other conditions of the lower respiratory tract that are suppurative or necrotic (J85-J86) include abscess with gangrene or necrosis and pyothorax.

There are several types of pleural effusion (J90-J91) including malignancy or heart failure but some of these require the use of other codes so be sure to check the exclude notes. Pleural effusion is the inflammation of the pleural cavity.

Pneumothorax and air leak (J93) is when air or gas is present in the pleural cavity oftentimes due to trauma. It can be spontaneous, primary, or secondary. In secondary pneumothorax, the underlying condition needs to be coded first. There are numerous types of pneumothorax that are excluded such as traumatic (S27.0), iatrogenic (J95) as caused by medical treatment. Spontaneous means the air is able to enter the pleural space but not leave it.

Section 15.11: INTRAOPERATIVE/POSTPROCEDURAL   Respiratory conditions that develop during or after a procedure has been performed are coded as J95 which can include tracheostomy complications, pulmonary insufficiency, chemical pneumonitis due to anesthesia, hemorrhage, hematoma, puncture, laceration, air leak, and complications from the use of a ventilator (respirator) for breathing.

Respiratory failure and insufficiency (J96) is the inability of the respiratory system to provide adequate levels of oxygen and to adequately remove carbon dioxide.

RESPIRATORY QUIZ 9

1. What are the codes for a patient with lower respiratory infection?

2. What are the codes for an asthmatic patient with status asthmaticus and COPD?

3. What are the codes for a patient with COPD and emphysema?

4. What are the codes for a patient with chronic respiratory failure and chronic edema?

5. What are the codes for a patient with ARDS?

6. What are the codes for a patient who is dehydrated and has pneumonia of the right lobe?

7. What are the codes for a patient with pleurisy due to TB?

8. What are the codes for a collapsed lung?

9. What are the codes for a patient with a sore throat?

10. What are the codes for a patient with tonsillitis and adenoiditis?

11. What are the codes for a patient who is seen today for a high fever and chest congestion due to the common cold?

12. What are the codes for a patient with COPD with pneumonia?

13. What are the codes for a patient with acute and chronic bronchitis and COPD?

14. What are the codes for a patient with chronic bronchitis and emphysema?

15. What are the codes for a patient with asthma that was precipitated by exercise?

CHAPTER 16
ICD-10 DIGESTIVE SYSTEM

You will learn the following objectives in this chapter:

A. Digestive System
B. Diseases of the Mouth
C. Diseases of Esophagus and Stomach
D. Diseases of the Appendix
E. Hernias
F. Enteritis/Colitis
G. Other Diseases of the Intestines
H. Diseases of the Peritoneum
I. Liver Diseases
J. Disorders of Gallbladder and Pancreas
K. Other Diseases of the Digestive System
L. Procedural Complications

Chapter 11 is described as "Diseases of the Digestive System" and ranges from K00-K95. Dental conditions are no longer coded in this chapter but have been moved to the musculoskeletal chapter. There are two new sections for liver diseases (K70-K77) and disorders of gallbladder, biliary tract and pancreas (K80-K87).

Section 16.1: THE DIGESTIVE SYSTEM

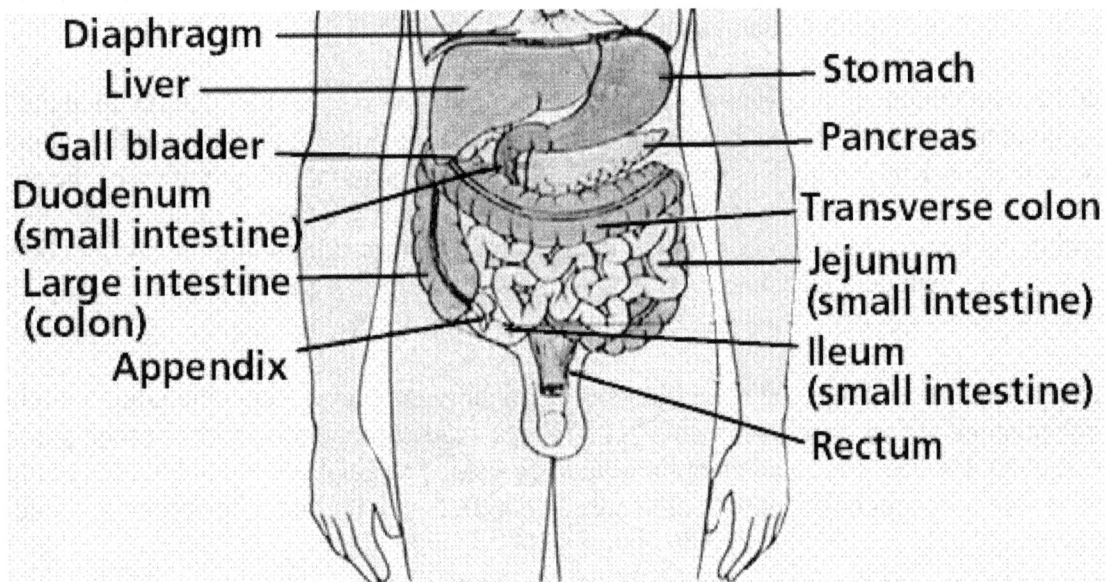

http://www.niddk.nih.gov/digesyst/digesyst.html.

The digestive system (also known as the gastrointestinal tract) includes from the top (mouth) to the bottom (anus).

The pharynx (throat), as discussed in the respiratory packet, extends from the mouth downwards where it separates into the trachea (windpipe) and the esophagus which is controlled by the epiglottis. It is through the esophagus that food travels into the stomach through contractions of muscles known as peristalsis.

The pyloric sphincter separates the stomach from the duodenum, which is the first part of the small intestine (small bowel). The next part of the small intestine is the jejunum, and then last is the ileum. Please note the spelling, ileum is part of the small intestine and should not be confused with the ilium.

From the ileum, the digestive system continues with the large intestine (large bowel) composed of the cecum, the colon (ascending colon, transverse colon, descending colon), then the sigmoid colon, and the rectum which terminates in the anus. The appendix hangs from the cecum.

Section 16.2: DISEASES OF THE MOUTH

This chapter contains many new notes that direct the coding of external causes, underlying conditions, and additional factors influencing the patient's condition, e.g. tobacco dependence (F17) and alcohol abuse and dependence (F10).

Alcohol and tobacco abuse are most oftentimes coded additionally as indicated in the notes for diseases in this chapter.

This section of codes begin with dental conditions and progress through the oral cavity and salivary glands (K00-K14). These include anodontia (K00.0) (absence of teeth), supernumerary teeth, disturbances in tooth formation and eruption, and teething (K00.4) in children.

The codes then continue into diseases of the hard tissues in the mouth (K02-K03) which includes caries, excessive wearing away of the teeth, abrasions and erosions. Conditions of the pulp and gum follow (K04-K08). This includes gingivitis which is a bacterial inflammation of the gums. Periodontitis is rapid onset of inflammation of the gums (gingiva) or peridontium (tissue supporting the teeth). Abnormalities of the dentofacial structures (including the jaw and bones follow next and include malocclusion (improper alignment of teeth and/or arches). Lastly, there are codes for other or unspecified conditions such as loss of teeth.

The codes then proceed into codes for diseases of the salivary glands (K11) including atrophy and sialoadenitis. Diseases of the mouth (K12-K13) include lips and oral mucosa such as abscess, cheilosis, cheek biting, leukoplakia, and fibrosis. The final section is diseases of the tongue (K14) which includes glossitis, hypertrophy, geographic tongue, plicated tongue, and glossodynia.

Section 16.3: DISEASES OF ESOPHAGUS, STOMACH & DUODENUM

Diseases of the esophagus and stomach (K20-K31) begin with disease of the esophagus and include esophagitis, ulcers, stricture, diverticulum, and laceration.

Reflux esophagitis (K21) is a similar condition to gastric esophageal reflux diseases (GERD), but it does not include the stomach. GERD is coded as K21 and includes the esophagus and stomach. It is caused by reflux of acidic stomach fluids up through the esophagus which can result in erosion of the esophagus.

Ulcers are lesions that form necrotic tissue due to inflammation which leaves a hole. Ulcers, again, are coded by what anatomic sites are involved, so the codes vary by anatomic site. Esophageal ulcers (lesion) are coded as K22.1 and are differentiated with or without bleeding. If drugs or poisonings are involved with the ulcer, then these should be coded also with T36-T65.

Gastric ulcers (K25) are also known as peptic ulcers that include the stomach and pylorus.

Duodenal ulcers (K26) are ulcers of the duodenum which is part of the small intestine. This is coded similar to gastric ulcers.   Previously peptic ulcers were listed under gastric ulcers although they are of the stomach so they are known as gastroduodenal ulcers.

Gastrojejunal ulcer (K28) occurs in both the stomach and jejunum but excludes primary ulcer of the small intestine as directed in the ICD-10 book.

For all of the ulcers, fourth characters further classify codes by being acute or chronic and with hemorrhage or perforation, e.g. chronic gastric ulcer with hemorrhage and perforation is coded as K25.6, but they are not classified as bleeding. Bleeding is only used to refer to gastritis, dudodenitis, diverticulosis and diverticulitis. The reference to obstruction has been eliminated.

Gastritis and duodenitis (K29) include acute, alcoholic, chronic as either superficial or atrophic, and unspecified as specified by the fourth digits. The fifth digits indicate if there is bleeding or not.

Other disease of the stomach and duodenum (K31) include dilatation of stomach, hypertrophic pyloric stenosis, hourglass stricture and stenosis of stomach, pylorospasm, fistula, and gastroparesis.

Diverticulum is a pouch or sac that can be acquired or genetic. Acquired means that the diverticulum was a result of an occurrence and that the person was not born with it (genetic). This can occur in various locations of the digestive tract, i.e. esophagus (K22.5), appendix (K38.2), and stomach (K31.4); these codes do not provide a description of inflammation (diverticulitis) or the abnormal condition of having diverticulum (diverticulosis) which are coded with K57 codes.

Section 16.4: DISEASES OF THE APPENDIX

Diseases of the appendix (K35-K38) include appendicitis which is inflammation of the appendix. This code is differentiated as including generalized or localized peritonitis (inflammation of the peritoneum). The peritonitis code includes appendicitis that also includes perforation or rupture. Other diseases of the appendix include hyperplasia, concretions, and fistula.

Section 16.5: HERNIAS

Hernias (K40-K46) are protrusions of any part of tissues and organs through an abnormal break in the muscular wall. A hiatal hernia is a hernia of the digestive system, specifically a protrusion of the stomach into the hernia. Inguinal hernia is a hernia of the groin area. An incisional hernia are hernias located at an incompletely-healed surgical wound. If the incisional hernia is in the stomach area, these are known as ventral hernias.

Both acquired and congenital hernias are coded from codes K40-K46 except for congenital diaphragmatic hernia (Q79.0) and congenital hiatus hernia (Q40.1). Like the ICD-9 codes, the hernias are coded as to site, e.g. inguinal, and are further specified in the fourth character as to the presence of obstruction and/or gangrene. Laterality and recurrence are also coded.

Obstructive hernias include hernias that are strangulated and incarcerated. A hernia is considered strangulated when the blood supply is compromised due to a constriction. A hernia is considered incarcerated when the bowels are completely obstructed.

Irreducible hernia is a hernia that cannot be returned to its original place.

An incomplete hernia has not completely gone through the break but in a complete hernia the protrusion has gone entirely through the opening.

Section 16.6: ENTERITIS & COLITIS

Noninfective enteritis and colitis (K50-K52) include Crohn's disease of the small or large intestines. Fifth characters indicate bleeding, obstruction, fistula or abscess. Manifestations should also be coded additionally.

Ulcerative colitis (K51) includes inflammation of the ileum (ileitis), rectosigmoid, and rectum (proctitis). It also includes inflammation of polyps in the colon. The fifth digit indicates bleeding, obstruction, fistula, abscess or other.

Other noninfective gastroenteritis and colitis (K52) can be due to radiation, allergy, dietary, or toxic adverse effects.

Section 16.7: OTHER DISEASES OF THE INTESTINES

Vascular disorders of the intestines (K55) include various types of colitis, infarction, ischemia, thrombosis, and angiodysplasia of the colon. Paralytic ileus and intestinal obstructions without hernia are coded as K56 which includes the bowel, colon and intestine. These codes include intussusception, volvulus, gallstones in the ileus, fecal impaction, and intestinal adhesions. Intussusception occurs when one section of the intestine collapses within another section. A volvulus is when the intestine twists upon itself.

Diverticular disease of intestines (K57) include diverticulitis and diverticular disease but diverticulum alone was previously coded in other sections. These codes arc differentiated with the fourth digit as to location and with or without perforation and abscess. The fifth digit indicates with or without bleeding.

Irritable bowel syndrome is coded as K58 with or without diarrhea.

Other intestinal disorders and diseases (K59-K63) include constipation, diarrhea, neurogenic bowel, anal spasm, megacolon, fissures, fistulas, abscess, polyp, stenosis, hemorrhage, ulcer and proctitis due to radiation. Anal fissures are cuts or tears in the tissue of the anus and anal fistulas are abnormal connections between the anus or rectum and the skin.

Hemorrhoids (K64) are dilated, swollen, painful veins in the anus or rectum. These can be complicated by thrombosis, bleeding, strangulation, ulceration, and prolapse (falling down or slipping out of place). They are classified by grades/stages from I to IV based on various factors such as bleeding, prolapse, and manual replacement. There are also hemorrhoidal skin tags and perianal venous thrombosis coded in this section.

Section 16.8: DISEASES OF PERITONEUM AND RETROPERITONEUM

Peritonitis (K65) is inflammation of the peritoneum. There are many excludes to these codes such as for various infections, foreign substances and neonatal. If peritonitis is coded from K65 then the infectious agent should also be coded, as would be with any infection. These peritonitis codes include generalize, spontaneous bacterial, abscess, sclerosing mesenteritis, and others.

Other disorders of the peritoneum (K66-K67) include for diseases classified elsewhere, adhesions and hemoperitoneum (traumatic coded as S36.8 instead).

Disorders of retroperitoneum (K68) include abscess including postprocedural.

Section 16.9: LIVER DISEASES

Diseases of the liver (K70-K77) are differentiated by cause such as alcohol or toxic substance. Fifth digits refer to the presence of various conditions such as ascites, sclerosis, fibrosis, hepatitis, cirrhosis, failure, cholestasis, and necrosis across the various causes.

Hepatitis can be persistent, lobular, active or other. Necrosis is death of the liver. Liver failure is differentiated as to with or without coma and as either acute, subacute or chronic.

Chronic liver disease leads to damage to the liver with cirrhosis and hepatitis. Cirrhosis is the destruction of liver cells and replacement of normal liver tissue with fatty tissue and can be caused by alcohol, malnutrition, or other conditions.

Other diseases that involve the liver (K76-K77) include fatty liver, congestion, hemorrhagic necrosis, infarction, occlusive disease, hepatorenal syndrome, and in diseases classified elsewhere.

Section 16.10: DISORDERS OF GALLBLADDER, BILIARY TRACT & PANCREAS

Cholecystitis and cholelithiasis are coded as K80 and now specify presence of cholangitis, e.g. calculus of bile duct with cholangitis (K80.3). Cholelithiasis (K80) is formation of calculus in the gallbladder and/or bile ducts, more commonly known as stones. These codes are differentiated as to whether acute or chronic cholecystitis is present or not. Cholecystitis is inflammation of the gallbladder and/or bile ducts and can be coded singly as K81.

Choledocholithiasis (K80.6) is obstruction of the common bile duct by calculus. Calculus of the bile ducts with cholangitis is coded as K80.3 and is differentiated as to being with or without obstruction and acute or chronic.

Other disease of the gallbladder (K82) include obstruction, hydrops, perforation, fistula, and cholesterolosis. Other diseases of the biliary tract (K83) include cholangitis, obstruction, perforation, fistula, cyst and spasm of sphincter of Oddi (SOD).

Acute pancreatitis and other diseases of the pancreas (K85-K86) can be idiopathic, biliary, alcohol or drug induced. Other diseases of the pancreas include alcohol-induced chronic pancreatitis or other cause, cyst, pseudocyst, and other such as necrosis and cirrhosis.

Section 16.11: OTHER DISEASES OF DIGESTIVE SYSTEM

Oftentimes, a person may be ingesting sufficient food but the body is not able to process the food which is known as malabsorption. Other diseases of the digestive system (K90-K95) include various diseases that affect the digestive process such as celiac disease, tropical sprue, blind loop syndrome, steatorrhea, malabsorption due to intolerance, and Whipple's disease. Celiac disease occurs when the stomach is coated by the gluten from grain products which then prevents the stomach from absorbing and distributing the food that is processed in the stomach. Steatorrhea occurs when there is the presence of excess fats in the stool due to the processing and malabsorption of fats.

GI hemorrhaging includes hematemesis (K92.0) which is spitting up blood and melena/hematochezia (K92.1) which is black tarry stools due to the presence of digested blood. Hematochezia is bright red blood in the stools. Vomiting blood and spitting blood are not the same diagnosis. Spitting blood is known as hemoptysis (R04.2).

Other diseases include ulcerative gastrointestinal mucositis (K92.8) with the need to code also if therapy such as for cancer was administered (T45.1X).

Section 16.12: INTRAOPERATIVE AND POSTPROCEDURAL

Complications and disorders associated with the digestive system due to medical procedures (intraoperative and postprocedural) (K91) include vomiting, dumping syndrome, postgastrectomy syndrome, malabsorption, obstruction, postcholecystectomy syndrome, hemorrhages, hematoma, puncture, laceration, hepatic failure, and pouchitis.

Complications from an artificial opening (K94), such as a stomy, include infections, hemorrhage, malfunction, and mechanical problems. Stomies for the digestive system include colostomy, enterostomy, gastrostomy, and esophagostomy. Complications from bariatric procedures (K95) such as gastric band procedures include infection or other complication. If the organism causing the infection is known it must also be coded.

DIGESTIVE QUIZ 10

1. What is the code for a patient diagnosed with a peptic ulcer?

2. What are the codes for a patient with a perforated appendix with an abscess?

3. What are the codes for a patient with Crohn's disease?

4. What are the codes for a patient with gastritis and duodenitis?

5. What is the code for GERD?

6. What are the codes for a patient with hemorrhagic alcoholic gastritis?

7. What are the codes for a patient with dysentery and gastritis due to Salmonella?

8. What are the codes for a patient with Crohn's disease of large and small intestines?

9. What are the codes for a patient with acute cholecystitis with bile duct calculus and obstruction?

10. What are the codes for a patient with volvulus with hernia of the intestine with gangrene?

11. What are the codes for a patient with postoperative hernia?

12. What are the codes for a patient with acute gastric ulcer?

13. What are the codes for a patient with gastritis due to alcoholism?

14. What are the codes for a patient with retropharyngeal abscess?

15. What are the codes for a patient with incarcerated inguinal hernia?

CHAPTER 17
ICD-10 INTEGUMENTARY SYSTEM

You will learn the following objectives in this chapter:

A. Integumentary System
B. Infections of the Skin
C. Dermatitis and Eczema
D. Urticaria and Erythema
E. Radiation
F. Disorders of Appendages
G. Other Disorders

Chapter 12 is described as "Diseases of the Skin and Subcutaneous Tissue" and ranges from L00-L99. Many conditions have been removed to other chapters so many changes have been made to this chapter as well as expansions of many codes. Greater specificity has also been added to many codes including a new section (block) for radiation-related disorders of the skin and subcutaneous tissue. There are also some terminology changes.

Section 17.1: INTEGUMENTARY SYSTEM

Integumentary is the skin and its accessory organs which include hair, nails and glands. It is the largest organ of the body. The purpose of the integumentary system is to provide protection, thermoregulation, sensation, and allows secretion. It also prevents the loss of water, salts, and other nutrients.

The first layer of the skin is known as the epidermis and is composed only of squamous epithelium cells. The dermis lies below the epidermis and is composed of blood and lymph vessels, nerve fibers, hair follicles, sweat glands, and the sebaceous glands which are connected through connective tissue. The subcutaneous layer is a layer of connective tissue and also aids in the formation and storage of fat in cells known as lipocytes.

Erythema is reddening of the skin. Ecchymosis is a bluish-black discoloration of the skin, such as a bruise, which occurs due to the loss of blood from its vessels. Petechiae are the same as ecchymosis but smaller. Purpura is when ecchymoses and petechiae grow larger and merge. Vitiligo is loss of pigment (melanin).

Skin neoplasms can be benign or malignant as previously discussed. Benign skin neoplasms include calluses, keloids, nevus, and verruca. A scar is also known as a cicatrix. Verruca are also known as warts and are caused by the human papillomavirus (HPV).

Section 17.2: INFECTIONS OF SKIN AND SUBCUTANEOUS TISSUE

Infections of skin and subcutaneous tissue section (L00-L08) begins with Staphylococcal scalded skin syndrome (L00). Percentage of skin exfoliated should be coded additionally (L49). It is also known as Ritter's disease and staphylococcal epidermal necrolysis. It involves blistering of the skin which results in exfoliation which can vary from a few blisters to affecting the entire body.

Erysipelas is a superficial infection of the skin which is coded as A46 in another section. Impetigo (L01) is a bacterial infection of the skin as evidenced by the presence of pustules and lesions.

Abscesses, furuncles, and carbuncles (L02) are painful bumps formed under the skin. A furuncle (boil) is an infection of the hair follicles. A carbuncle is a composite of several furuncles and is an abscess with pus that is larger and most often due to a bacterial infection. While many anatomic sites are included in this section, there are many exclusions because they are coded in other sections specific to the anatomic site, such as the ear, mouth and nose.

If the organism causing the infection is known it should also be coded. In this section, the anatomic sites coded include face, neck, trunk, buttock, limb, hand, foot, and other sites not listed elsewhere.

An infection of the skin is known as cellulitis (L03) which extends into the subcutaneous tissues and can lead to further sepsis if not treated properly. Lymphangitis (inflammation of the lymph system) is also included in this section. There are many exclusions in this section based on anatomic site such as breast.

Lymphadenitis (L04) is inflammation of the lymph nodes except mesenteric. This is differentiated by anatomic site such as face, head, neck, trunk, and limbs.

Lesions are damaged tissue. There are many types of lesions depending on their appearance and condition. A macule is a discolored flat lesion. This includes freckles and moles. A prominence above the skin would include cyst, polyp, pustule, vesicle, nodule, papule, and wheal.

Pilonidal cysts (L05) are cysts in the buttock area and coded with or without abscess and including sinus or not. Other local infections (L08) include pyoderma.

Bullous disorders (L10-L14) include Pemphigus (L10) which is a chronic autoimmune disease in which blisters appear. There are several types of pemphigus which includes vulgaris, vegetans, follaceous, Brazilian and drug-induced. Pemphigoid (L12) resembles pemphigus in that there are large blisters too. It can be caused by drugs or can be bullous or cicatrical. Other bullous disorders include dermatitis herpetiformis.

Section 17.3: DERMATITIS AND ECZEMA

Dermititis and eczema are terms used interchangeably and are coded as L20-L30. Again, sometimes these conditions are coded in other sections based on anatomic site.

There are many types of dermatitis and it can be due to many things, including contact dermatitis (L23-L27) which includes exposure to various agents such as metals, adhesives, cosmetics, dyes, cement, insecticide, plastic, rubber, and animal dander. Contact dermatitis can also be described as being due to irritants such as detergents, drugs, and solvents which may also be taken internally.

Pruritus (L29) which is itching. Eczemas coded as other specified dermatitis (L30) and is inflammation of the skin and may be accompanied by pruritus and formation of lesions.

Papulosquamous disorders (L40-L45) include psoriasis (L40) which is a skin condition characterized by itchy reddened scales. It also includes lichen planus which is an itchy rash on the skin. Psoriasis (L40.5) is an autoimmune disease that appears as red scaly patches on the skin, fingernails, and toenails. The most common type is plaque psoriasis. Psoriasis has been expanded to include manifestations, e.g. psoriatic arthritis mutilans (L40.52).

Section 17.4: URTICARIA AND ERYTHEMA

Urticaria and erythema are coded as L49-L54. Included in this section are codes for exfoliation which can result from erythema and which requires that the condition causing the exfoliation be coded first such as Stevens-Johnson Syndrome. These codes are based on percentage of body affected. Exfoliation (L49) is oftentimes coded with the etiological condition.

Urticaria (L50) is red wheals on the skin due to allergic reactions and are also known as hives. Urticaria can be allergic, idiopathic, dermatographic, vibratory, cholinergic or contact related.

Erythema (L51-L53) is classified as toxic, multiforme, nodosum, rosacea, and lupus. Additional codes should be coded for manifestations such as arthropathy, edema, ulcers, and stomatitis. Toxic erythema is a common rash caused by poisonings, so the drug or toxin should be listed if known. Erythema multiforme can be a minor or major red rash. The most severe form is known as Stevens-Johnson syndrome. Erythema nodosum is an inflammation of the fat cells under the skin (panniculitis).

Section 17.5: RADIATION

Radiation-related disorders (L55-L59) include sunburns (L55) with fourth characters classifying if the burn was first, second, or third degree.

Other radiation-related skin disorders include drug response, solar urticarial, chronic exposure to nonionizing radiation, actinic keratosis (pre-malignant condition of thick scaly skin patches), and radiodermatitis. The source of radiation should also be coded (W89).

Section 17.6: DISORDERS OF THE APPENDAGES

Disorders of the appendages (L60-L75) includes nails. This includes ingrown toenails (L60).

Various types of hair loss are coded in this section including alopecia which is the loss of hair from areas where hair should be, such as the top of the head. It can be due to hereditary conditions, medications, toxins, or trauma. There is a code for male-pattern baldness (androgenic, L64).   Hair coloring and hair shaft abnormalities include premature greying. Hypertrichosis includes hirsutism which is excessive hair growth where there normally would not be.

Acne (L70) forms from the buildup of sebum and keratin from the skin in the pores which causes a blockage. It is also known as acne vulgaris. Partial blockage is known as a comedone (blackhead) and complete blockage is known as a whitehead because there is also the collection of the pus. Seborrhea is a scaly, flaky itchy, red skin disorder affecting the scalp, face, and trunk, known as dandruff on the scalp but it is coded as L21.0 and is not in this section.

Rosacea (L71) is facial erythema with inflammation.

Follicular disorders include cysts including a sebaceous cyst (L72.3), acne keloid and eccrine or apocrine sweat disorders. Anhidrosis (L74.4) is the inability of the body to sweat. If a person sweats too much this is known as hyperhidrosis (L74.5).

Intraoperative and postoperative complications are coded as L76 and include hemorrhage, hematoma, puncture, and laceration.

Section 17.7: OTHER DISORDERS

Other disorders (L80-L99) include vitiligo which involves depigmentation of parts of the skin. Other disorders of pigmentation include freckles, café au lait spots, cholasma, and tattoo pigmentation.

Seborrheic keratosis can be either inflamed or other. Corns and callouses are coded as L84. Epidermal thickening (L85) includes ichthyosis and xerosis cutis or dry skin dermatitis.

A break in the skin can occur from a fissure, erosion, or ulcer. Pressure ulcers, which include decubitus ulcers, are coded as L89 and include many sites. Non-pressure ulcers are coded as L97. Decubitus ulcers, commonly known as bedsores, occur when there is continuous pressure on a portion of a skin in the buttock area which results in a breakdown of the skin. Ulcer codes have been expanded significantly with fourth characters indicating the specific site and fifth characters specifying the breakdown of the skin (fat layer exposed, necrosis, and unspecified). The sixth character indicates the stage of the progression of the disease of the ulcer from Stage 1 to Stage 4 which involves necrosis.

INTEGUMENTARY QUIZ 11

1) What are the codes for a patient with severe dermatitis due to her use of pierced earrings?

2) What are the codes for a patient with infected corn on the right big toe with cellulitis with possible sepsis and COPD with diabetes?

3) What are the codes for a 2-month-old baby who presents with a diaper rash?

4) What are the codes for a patient with nonbullous erythema multiforme?

5) What are the codes for a patient with second degree sunburn?

6) What are the codes for a patient with exfoliation on 34% of their body due to erythema multiforme with arthropathy?

7) What are the codes for a patient with pilonidal cyst with abscess?

8) What are the codes for a patient with cheloid scar after an appendectomy?

9) What are the codes for a patient with impetiginous dermatitis?

10) What are the codes for a patient with impetigo simplex?

11) What are the codes for a patient with albinism?

12) What are the codes for a patient with winter's itch?

13) What are the codes for a patient with dermatitis due to allergy to dust?

14) What are the codes for a patient with a stage 2 ulcer that developed from a cast that was applied to their right lower leg for 3 months due to a fracture?

15) What are the codes for a patient with chronic lymphangitis due to staph?

CHAPTER 18
ICD-10 MUSCULOSKELETAL SYSTEM

You will learn the following objectives in this chapter:

A. Musculoskeletal Anatomy
      1. Bones
      2. Muscles
      3. Joints
B. Arthropathies
      1. Pyogenic Arthritis
      2. Crystal Arthropathies
      3. Rheumatoid Arthritis
      4. Juvenile Rheumatoid Arthritis
      5. Osteoarthritis
      6. Other Arthritis
      7. Derangement
      8. Rheumatism
C. Dentofacial
D. Connective Tissue Disorders
E. Dorsopathies
F. Spondylopathies
G. Soft Tissue Disorders
H. Disorders of Synovium and Tendon
I. Osteopathies and Chondropathies
J. Procedural Complications
K. Biomechanical Lesions

Chapter 13 is described as "Diseases of the Musculoskeletal System and Connective Tissue" and ranges from M00-M99. There are many changes, deletions, expansions, and moves within this chapter with almost every code having been changed in some way including designation of laterality.

Section 18.1: MUSCULOSKELETAL ANATOMY

The musculoskeletal system includes the bones, muscles, and joints. Connective tissue includes bones, cartilage, and fibrous tissue. It also includes blood and fat. Bones are organs and are the framework for the body that gives it support, protects the internal organs, and assist in movement.

The middle part of the bone (not to be confused with the inside of the bone) is known as the shaft and is called the diaphysis. The ends of the bone are known as the epiphysis. There is an epiphyseal plate in the bone where the growth occurs which is of importance in the growth of children. The bone is covered by the periosteum.

Cranial bones are the bones of the skull (cranium) and protect the brain. The frontal bone is at the front of the head. Parietal bones (two) are on each side of the skull. Temporal bones (two) are on the lower sides and base of the skull. Occipital bone is at the back and base of the skull. Sphenoid bone is located behind the eyes. Ethmoid bone is behind the nose.

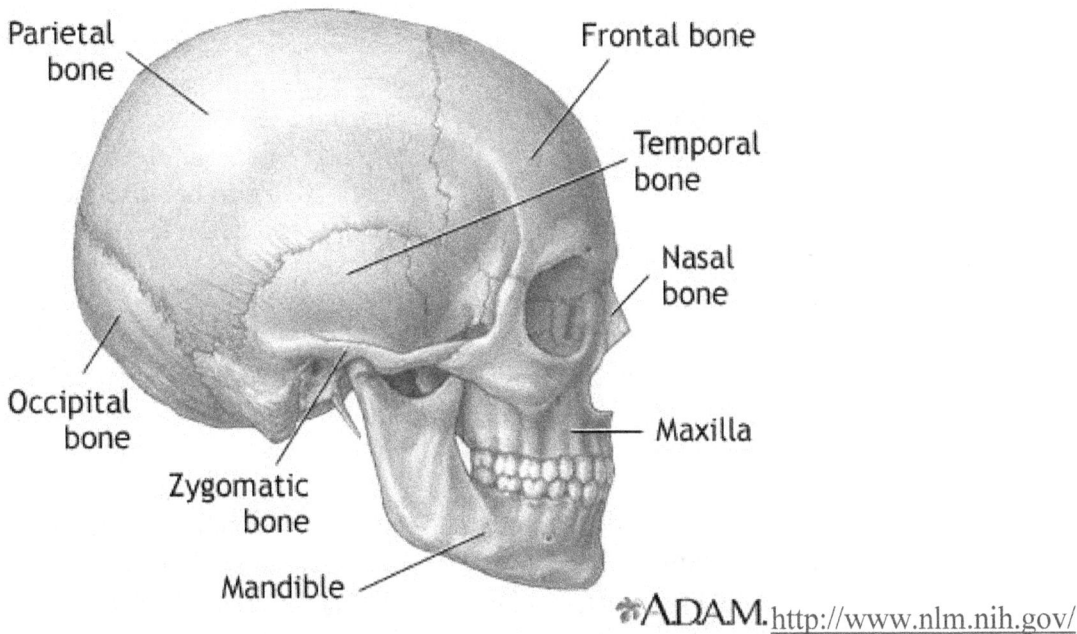

ADAM. http://www.nlm.nih.gov/

FACIAL: Facial bones include two nasal bones, two lacrimal bones (corner of each eye), two zygomatics (cheeks), vomer (lower part of the nose), two maxillary (upper jaw), and the mandible (lower jaw). The sinuses are located within these areas including the frontal, ethmoidal, sphenoidal, and maxillary sinuses.

SPINE: The bones protecting the spinal cord are known as the spinal column or vertebrae. The vertebrae are separated by cartilage known as intervertebral disks. The spine is divided into five divisions: 7 cervical vertebrae (neck, C1-C7), 12 thoracic (chest & ribs, T1-T12), 5 lumbar (lower back, L1-L5), 1 sacrum, and 1 coccyx (tailbone).

The posterior part of the veterbrae is composed of the vertebral arch, spinous process, 2 transverse processes, and 2 laminae.

Nih.gov

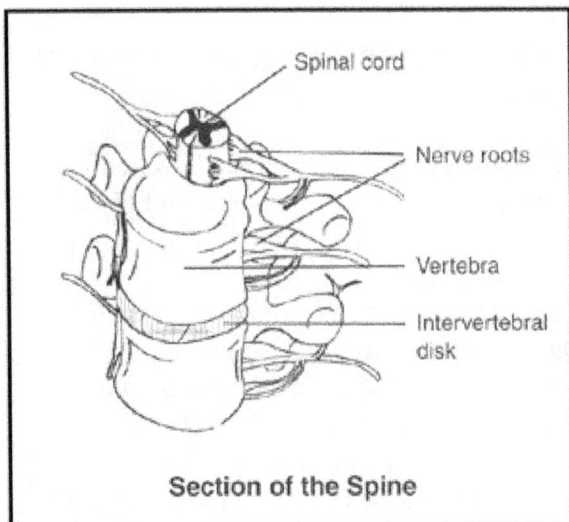

Section of the Spine

Carpals

Metacarpals

Phalanges

Tarsals

Metatarsals

Phalanges

Skull
Clavicle
Scapula
Sternum
Rib
Humerus
Vertebrae
Ulna
Radius
Sacrum
Femur
Patella
Tibia
Fibula

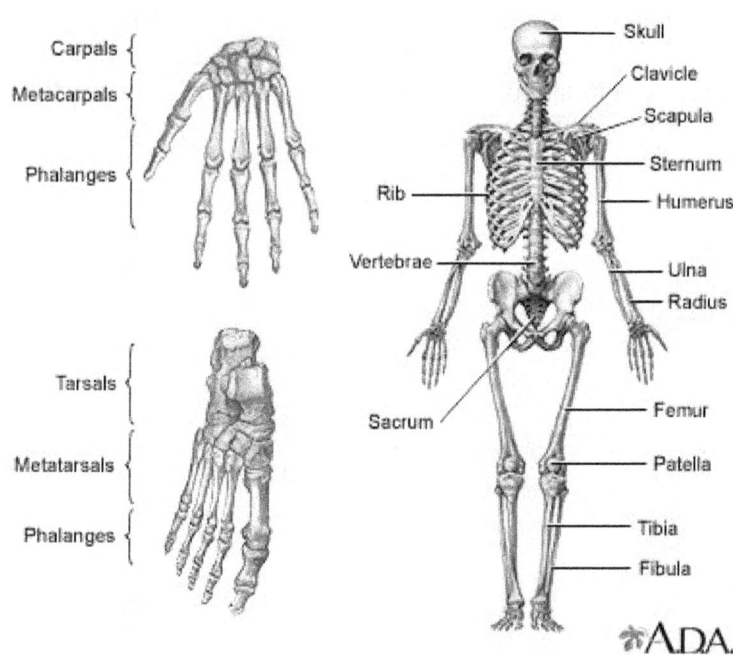

TRUNK: Bones of the trunk include the clavicle (collar bone), scapula (shoulder blade), sternum (breastbone), and ribs (12 pairs).

RIBS: Ribs 8 to 10 are known as the false ribs because they attach posteriorly with the 7th rib and ribs 11 and 12 are known as the floating ribs because they are not attached in the front.

PELVIS: Bones of the pelvis include the pelvic girdle (composed of the ilium, pubis, and ischium).

✱A.D.A.M. Nih.gov

EXTREMITIES: The bones of the arms include the humerus (upper), ulna (medial lower which includes the olecranon which is better known as the elbow), radius (lateral lower in line with the thumb), carpals (wrist bones), metacarpals (palm), and phalanges (fingers). The phalanges have three segments, proximal, middle, and distal. The proximal are closest to the palm. For the phalanges, PIP are proximal interphalangeal joints between the first (also called proximal) and second (intermediate) phalanges. DIP are distal interphalangeal joints between the second and third (distal) phalanges.

The bones of the legs include the femur (thigh bone), patella (knee cap), tibia (largest of lower leg bones on the inside), fibula (smallest of lower leg bones on the outside), tarsals (back of foot composed of the calcaneus, heel bone and talus), metatarsals (midfoot), and phalanges (toes).

The femur is the longest bone in the body and its acetabulum fits into the socket of the pelvic girdle.

MUSCLES: Muscles are responsible for movement which consists of contractions and relaxation. There are over 600 muscles. They can be attached to bones, organs, and blood vessels.

There are three types of muscles: striated, smooth, and cardiac. Striated muscles are voluntary (skeletal) muscles. They move the bones and are consciously controlled. Smooth muscles are involuntary (visceral) muscles. They move the internal organs and are controlled by the autonomic nervous system. Cardiac muscles are the muscles of the heart.

A muscle can extend or flex. Flexion is a muscle movement in which the angle between the bones is decreased (bending). Extension is a muscle movement in which the angle between the bones is increased (straightening out). Dorsiflexion is the decreasing of the angle of the ankle joint. Plantar flexion is the increasing of the angle of the ankle joint (pointing of toes).

A muscle can move away from the midline of the body (abduction) or move towards the midline of the body (adduction).

Rotation is circular turning. Supination if the turning of the palm up and pronation is the turning of the palm down.

JOINTS: Joints are the attachment point where bones come together which is known as articulation. The ends of the bones are covered with the articular cartilage so that the bones do not come directly together, otherwise this would be very painful to have bones rubbing on each other. The articular cartilage provides a cushion for the joint to move painlessly and smoothly.

Joints can be movable or immovable. Joints that are immovable include the suture joints of the skull. Joints that are very movable are known as synovial joints which include the ball-and-socket and hinge type. Movable joints include the knee and spine. Synovial joints are surrounded by fibrous tissues known as the joint capsule. The synovial fluid and membrane within it constitute the bursa (bursae).

LIGAMENTS: Ligaments (connective tissue) anchor the bones together. While ligaments connect bones together, tendons connect muscles to bones.

Rheumatism include disorders of the muscles and tendons and their attachments. Enthesopathies are disorders of the peripheral ligamentous or muscular attachments.

Section 18.2: ARTHOPATHIES

Arthropathies (M00-M25) include many types of arthropathies and arthritis. Arthritis is inflammation of the joints which can lead to joint pain, stiffness, and swelling to the point that it becomes difficult to do anything. Arthropathies/arthritis codes specify manifestations, sites, and laterality with the fourth, fifth and sixth characters.

Infectious arthropathies are coded as M00-M02. Infectious arthropathies can be either direct or indirect infections. Indirect infections can be either reactive or postinfective. Reactive arthropathies is when there was infection by an organism but it could not be identified.

Pyogenic (producing pus)/septic arthritis (M00) is caused by an infection such as staph, pneuomococcal or strep. If arthritis develops from an infection, then the codes for organism should also be coded.

Postinfective and reactive arthropathies are coded as M02 with a note to code first the underlying disease such as hepatitis. These arthropathies can occur after intestinal bypass, dysentery, immunization, and Reiter's disease.

Inflammatory polyarthropathies (M05-M14) include rheumatoid arthritis (RA). This is a chronic debilitating autoimmune disease of the joints. Scarring can occur on the bones which then can lead to ankylosis (stiffness of a joint that may result in bones fusing together, making movement difficult and painful) so that movement becomes painful and highly limited. Manifestations, such as myopathy or polyneuropathy, should be coded additionally as indicated in the codes. Notice that rheumatoid arthritis of the spine and rheumatic fever should be coded with codes from other sections as indicated in the codes.

Juvenile rheumatoid arthritis (JRA) (M08) begins before a person is 16 years old. The codes are distinguished as polyarticular, pauciarticular and monoartiuclar. Oligoarticular (pauciarticular) JRA affect four or fewer joints. Polyarticular JRA affects five or more joints. Monoarticular JRA affects one joint.

Crystal arthropathies (M1A) result from an accumulation of crystals in the joints. The accumulation of crystals in joints can be caused by gout which is caused by deposition of uric acid crystals in the joint, causing inflammation and is now included in these codes for arthropathies. High uric acid levels are related to gout. Gout conditions can be idiopathic (origin unknown), drug-induced, lead-induced, with renal impairment, as well as being secondary to other conditions such as myeloma and anemia. Other crystal arthropathies include hydroxyapatite deposition disease and familial chondrocalcinosis.

Other types of arthropathies include Felty's syndrome, lung disease, vasculitis, heart disease, myopathy, polyneuropathy, bursitis, nodules, enteropathies (digestive system disorders), and involvement of various organs, with or without organ involvement, Kaschin-Beck disease, villonodular synovitis, palindromic, transient, allergic, traumatic, and in other diseases such as Charcot's joint. .

Many of these codes have six characters. There is a seventh character for some of the codes such as M1A which is based on whether there is tophus or not present. Some of the codes require additional codes for other conditions present such as calculus and cardiomyopathy.

Gout has been expanded significantly (M1A) and has an unusual combination of letters and numbers for codes. It is differentiated by cause, laterality, etiology, anatomic site, and acute or chronic.

OSTEOARTHRITIS: Osteoarthritis (M15-M19) is inflammation of the bones and joints with erosion of cartilage and is also known as degenerative joint disease. This results in bone rubbing on bone. The most common form of arthritis, osteoarthritis (degenerative joint disease), is a result of trauma or other similar condition to the joint, infection of the joint, or age. Osteoarthritis is further specified by fourth characters for type (e.g. polyosteoarthritis) and fifth characters for laterality.

Polyosteoarthritis occurs in multiple sites. Post-traumatic osteoarthritis occurs after trauma (M19.1). Primary osteoarthritis is a chronic degenerative disorder related to but not caused by aging. Secondary osteoarthritis is caused by another condition, such as an infection or trauma. Localized osteoarthritis affects only the one site where it is located, while generalized affects multiple sites.

Section 18.3: OTHER JOINT DISORDERS

Other joint disorders (M20-M25) include acquired deformities although some deformities are coded in other sections as noted in the exclude note.

Deformities of fingers include mallet finger, Boutonniere, and Swan-neck.

Deformities of the feet include hallux valgus, otherwise known as a bunion. A bunion is a deformity of the bones and the joint between the foot and big toe caused by a swollen bursae and/or a bone deformity on the joint known as the medial eminence. Hallux valgus is when the big toe points away from the rest of the toes and is also commonly called a bunion. Hallux rigidus is a deformity of the great toe that causes pain upon flexion which limits motion.

Hammer toe is a deformity of the proximal interphalangeal joint of the second, third, or fourth toe causing it to be permanently bent. Claw toe is when a toe is contracted at the PIP and DIP joints (middle and end joints in the toe) which can lead to severe pressure and pain.

There are also wrist and foot drop and flat foot. If a person is flat-footed, that is coded as talipes planus

Similar deformities can occur in other anatomic sites, such as valgus and varus of the forearm (wrist, elbow, hand, etc.). Club hand is when the axis of the wrist is permanently deviated and the hand is usually closed.

Unequal limb lengths are specified by anatomic site of the arms and legs and by laterality.

Conditions of the patella are highly differentiated including dislocation, subluxation (partial dislocation), involving the femur, derangements, involving chondromalacia (softening of cartilage).

Internal derangement of the knee refers to disorders involving disruption of the normal functioning of the ligaments or cartilages (menisci) of the knee joint. Derangement of the knee (M23) includes degeneration, loose bodies in the traumatized area, softening, tear, or rupture of cartilage or meniscus of the knee, including an old bucket tear.

There are various disorders of the ligaments including spontaneous disruption, instability, and laxity. Dislocation of joints due to other diseases (pathological) is coded as M24.3 and differentiated by anatomic site and laterality. Dislocation of joints can also be recurrent. Other conditions of the joins include contracture, ankylosis (stiffness and immobility of joint with possible bone fusion), hemarthrosis (bleeding into joint space), fistula, flail (loss of function of joint due to destabilization), effusion, pain, stiffness, and osteophyte (bone spurs).

Section 18.4: DENTOFACIAL

Dentofacial anomalies (M26-M27) include various anomalies associated with teeth and the jaw such as malocclusion of the maxillae or mandible, macrogenia, microgenia, excessive tuberosity, asymmetry, reverse articulation, abnormal jaw closure, deviation in opening and closing of mandible, insufficient guidance, arthralgia, articular disc disorder, and excessive horizontal overlap. Anomalies of the teeth include crowding, excessive spacing, displacement, rotation, and insufficient distance between teeth.

Other diseases of the jaws include Torus palatinus, Giant cell granuloma, Stafne's cyst, osteitis, periostitis, sequestrum, cysts, overfill, and osseointegration failure of dental implant. Periostitis (M27.2) is inflammation of the periosteum which is the connective tissue surrounding bone.

Section 18.5: CONNECTIVE TISSUE DISORDERS

Connective tissue (mainly composed of collagen) exists in many anatomic sites, so diseases related to them can be found in differing sections of the coding book. Systemic connective tissue disorders (M30-M36) include polyarteritis nodosa, juvenile polyarteritis, Kawasaki's syndrome, granuloma, polyangiitis, and systemic lupus erythematosus (SLE).

SLE is an autoimmune disease wherein the body's immune system turns against itself. Sclerosis is the building up of scar tissue on connective tissue. Scleroderma is systemic sclerosis. Other systemic disorders of connective tissue include Sicca, Sjogren, Behcet, and panniculitis. Additional complications need to also be coded as indicated in the notation under these codes, as well as etiology if known.

Section 18.6: DORSOPATHIES

Dorsopathies (M40-M54) are disorders of the back. This section has been greatly enhanced based on etiology, anatomic site, and type. Various curvatures of the spine include kyphosis (curving that causes bowing like with a hunchback), lordosis (inward curvature) and flatback syndrome. Scoliosis is the curvature of spine from side to side. It can be infantile or juvenile idiopathic, thoracogenic, neuromuscular, or secondary. Torticollis is wry neck which is when the head tilts toward one side, and the chin is elevated and turned toward the opposite side.

Osteochondroses are conditions that affect the growth of the skeleton in that it is a disease that includes both the bone and cartilage bone and is characterized by interruption of the blood supply to the bone.

Section 18.7: SPONDYLOPATHIES

Spondylolysis is osteoarthritis of the vertebrae. Spondylolisthesis involves displacement of the vertebrae so it is classified by section of the spine involved. Spondylopathies (M45-M49) include ankylosing spondylitis which occurs when there is stiffness with possible fusion of the vertebrae which includes rheumatoid arthritis of the spine. Inflammatory spondylopathies include enthesopathy (disorder of bone attachments), osteomyelitis, infection, and discitis which all involve the spine. Spondylosis with radiculopathy and myelopathy are coded as M47.0 - M47.2.

Other spondylopathies include spinal stenosis, ankylosing hypoerostosis, kissing spine (condition in which the spinous processes of adjacent vertebra are touching, also known as Baastrup's disease or syndrome), traumatic, collapsed, and fatigue fracture of vertebrae but not pathological fracture which is coded as M84. There is a seventh character for collapsed and fatigue fracture for the type of encounter such as initial, subsequent, and sequel.

Spondylopathies in other diseases (M49) include various curvatures of the spine (e.g. kyphosis and scoliosis) due to other disease such as brucellosis which should be coded first.

Other dorsopathies (M50-M54) include cervical disc disorders with various other conditions such as myelopathy, radiculopathy, disc displacement, disc degeneration, and spinal instabilities. Dorsalgia is back and neck pain including panniculitis (inflammation of tissue beneath the skin), radiculopathy, sciatica (pain that starts in the sciatica nerve and goes down the leg), lumbago (pain in the lumbar region), low back pain, and backache.

Section 18.8: SOFT TISSUE DISORDERS

Soft tissue disorders of the muscles (M60-M63) include myositis (inflammation of the muscles) which can be infective or interstitial. Foreign bodies can produce granulomas (M60.2).

Calcifications and ossification of the muscles can occur known as myositis ossificans and can be traumatic or progressive. Calcification and ossification can occur with quadriplegia or paraplegia (M61.2). It can also be associated with burns.

Other disorders of the muscles include separation, rupture, and ischemic infarction of muscle nontraumatically (M62). These codes also include contracture of muscle and muscle wasting and atrophy.

Other diseases can also cause disorders of the muscles such as leprosy or neoplasm and are coded with M63 with a code for the disease coded first.

Section 18.9: DISORDERS OF SYNOVIUM AND TENDON

Disorders of the synovium and tendon (M65-M67) include synovitis and tenosynovitis which can involve abscesses, other infection, calcific tendinitis, and trigger finger (M65.3) which is stenosing tenosynovitis. This occurs when the motion of the tendon that opens and closes the finger is limited which causes the finger to lock or catch as the finger is extended.

Spontaneous rupture of the synovium or flexor/extensor tendons as well as other tendons is coded as M66. Rupture of the Achilles' tendon is coded as M67.0.

Other abnormal conditions of the synovium and tendons include hypertrophy, transient, toxic, ganglions (swelling or tumor on joint or tendon), and Plica syndrome (irritation to synovial tissues of the knee).

Other soft tissue disorders (M70-M79) include crepitant synovitis, and various bursitis. Bursitis is inflammation of the bursae which are the fluid-filled sacs around the joints caused oftentimes by repeated irritation or injury to the same location. Other disorders include conditions due to overuse and pressure. Abscesses and infections of bursa are coded with M71 and the organism causing it should also be coded. Synovial cysts of the popliteal space in the knee is also known as Baker's (M71.20). Other conditions of the bursa include other cysts, calcium deposits and other bursopathies.

Fibroblastic disorders (M72) include Dupuytren's Syndrome, knuckle pads, necrotizing fasciitis, and fibromatosis. Plantar fasciitis is inflammation of the foot caused by excessive wear to the plantar fascia that supports the arches of the foot. Dupuytren's disease is fasciitis of the hand which causes the fingers to bend in towards the palm. Necrotizing fasciitis (flesh-eating bacterial disease) is a rare infection of the deeper layers of skin and subcutaneous tissues. The organism should also be coded as indicated in the codes.

There is a section specific to lesions of the shoulder (M75) which includes adhesive capsulitis, rotator cuff tear or rupture (either incomplete or complete), tendinitis (either bicipital or calcific), impingement, and bursitis. .

Enthesopathies (M76-M77) include tendinitis of various anatomic sites such as gluteal, psoas, and iliac as well as epicondylitis (medial or lateral), periarthritis, calcaneal spur, and metatarsalgia. Lateral epicondylitis is also known as tennis elbow and golfer's elbow is medial epicondylitis). An epicondyle is a prominence on the distal part of a long bone serving as the attachment for muscles and ligaments.

Other soft tissue disorders (M79) include unspecified rheumatism, myalgia, residual foreign body, hypertrophy of fat pad, pain, fibromyalgia, and nontraumatic compartment syndrome. neuralgia, neuritis, and panniculitis which is inflammation of subcutaneous adipose (fatty) tissue. Compartment syndrome that is nontraumatic is caused by repetitive and extensive muscle use. This results in increased pressure due most frequently to inflammation within a confined space of the body, such as the lower leg which then impairs blood flow. Compartment syndrome that is traumatic would be coded as T79 as indicated in the codes. A nontraumatic seroma is a collection of fluid in soft tissue and nontraumatic hematoma is a collection of blood in soft tissue.

Section 18.10: OSTEOPATHIES AND CHONDROPATHIES

Osteopathies and chondropathies (M80-M94) include disorders of bone density and structure (M80-M85).

OSTEOPATHIES: Osteoporosis is a disease condition in which the bone mineral density (BMD) is reduced which can result in a greater susceptibility to bone fractures. Various types of osteoporosis include pathological (disease-caused) fracture which requires additional coding of the related osseous defect if known. Osteoporosis can also be age-related, drug-induced, idiopathic, from disuse, post surgical and post traumatic. Age-related (senile) osteoporosis is due to old age. In idiopathic osteoporosis the cause is not known. In disuse osteoporosis the cause is the lack of exercise and movement to utilize the bones.

If there was a previous fracture which has healed, a personal history code should be listed (Z87.310).

Seventh characters are required which designate type of encounter as initial, subsequent or sequela which are:

- A Initial encounter for closed fracture
- D Subsequent encounter for fracture with routine healing
- G Subsequent encounter for fracture with delayed healing
- K Subsequent encounter for fracture with nonunion
- P Subsequent encounter for fracture with malunion
- Q sequela

Softening of the bones is known as osteomalacia (M83) which can occur as an adult including puerperal, senile, due to malabsorption, malnutrition, aluminum bone disease or drug induced.

Other disorders of bones include discontinuity such as stress fractures (M84) such as fatigue, March, and stress.   Stress fractures are incomplete fracture in bones caused by unusual or repeated stress to the bone and can occur in various anatomic sites. The cause of the fracture should also be coded, if known.

Pathological fractures (M84.4) are fractures caused by a disease process and not from trauma. They can occur from a variety of conditions including chronic fatigue, neoplastic disease, and other diseases. The disease condition that caused the fracture should also be coded. All of these codes have seventh characters which are the same as previously discussed for osteoporosis.

Other disorders of bone density and structure include fibrous dysplasia, skeletal fibrosis, osteitis condensan, bone cysts, and acquired osteosclerosis.

Other osteopathies (M86-M90) include osteomyelitis (acute, subacute or various types of chronic) which is the inflammation and infection of the bone and/or bone marrow.

Osteonecrosis (M87) can be idiopathic aseptic, due to drugs, previous trauma, or secondary. It occurs when the bone does not get blood and dies.

Osteitis deformans (M88) include Paget's Disease which is a chronic disorder with excessive breakdown and formation of bone tissue that results in enlarged and deformed bones.

Other disorders of bones (M89) include algoneurodystrophy, physeal arrest (e.g. arrest of growth plate), hypertrophy, osteoarthropathy, and osteolysis. Osteolysis is breakdown (degeneration or dissolution) of bone.

Various diseases can cause osteopathies such as polio (M89.6) and rickets (M90.8) which require a code for the condition to also be listed.

CHONDROPATHIES: Chondropathies (M91-M94) are disease conditions of cartilage. This includes juvenile osteochrondrosis, nontraumatic slipped femoral epiphysis, osteochondritis dissecans, chondromalacia, and chondrolysis.

Other disorders of the musculoskeletal system and connective tissue (M95) include acquired deformities such as cauliflower ear.

Section 18.11: PROCEDURAL COMPLICATIONS AND DISORDERS

Intraoperative and postprocedural complications and disorders (M96) include pseudarthrosis after fusion or arthrodesis (fixation of joints), kyphosis, lordosis, scoliosis, postlaminectomy syndrome (continued numbness, tingling and muscle weakness), fracture of bone following insertion of implant, prosthesis or bone plate, hemorrhage, hematoma, puncture, and laceration.

Section 18.12: BIOMECHANICAL LESIONS

Biomechanical lesions (M99) include segmental and somatic dysfunction, subluxation, osseous or connective stenosis or lesions. These codes should not be used if the condition can be classified elsewhere.

MUSCULOSKELETAL QUIZ 12

1) What are the codes for a patient who has traumatic asphyxiation?

2) What are the codes for a patient who has pathological fracture of the vertebra due to osteoporosis?

3) What are the codes for a patient who has SLE with chronic nephritis?

4) What are the codes for a patient who has Achilles tenosynovitis?

5) What are the codes for a patient who has pyogenic arthritis of the hip due to staph?

6) What are the codes for a patient who has nonunion nondisplaced neck fracture of the left radius?

7) What are the codes for a patient who has degenerative joint disease of the knee?

8) What are the codes for a patient who has chronic obstructive asthma and neuropathy due to Type 2 diabetes which required treatment with insulin because it was uncontrolled?

9) What are the codes for a patient who has old bucket tear of the lateral meniscus of the right knee?

10) What are the codes for a patient who has a bone spur?

11) What are the codes for a patient who has acute osteomyelitis of the right ankle and foot?

12) What are the codes for a patient who has osteopathy due to typhoid fever?

13) What are the codes for a patient who has rheumatic polyarthritis with myopathy?

14) What are the codes for a patient who has carpal tunnel syndrome of the left arm?

15) What are the codes for a patient who has Sjogren's disease?

CHAPTER 19
ICD-10 GENITOURINARY SYSTEM

You will learn the following objectives in this chapter:

A. Genitourinary Systems
B. Glomerular Diseases
      1. Nephritis
      2. Glomerulonephritis
C. Renal Failure Disease
D. Urolithiasis
E. Other Diseases of Urinary System
F. Diseases of Male Genital Organs
      1. Benign Prostatic Hypertrophy
      2. Other Diseases
G. Breast Disorders
H. Disease of Female Genital Organs
      1. Gynecologic Disorders

Chapter 14 is described as "Diseases of the Genitourinary System" and ranges from N00-N99.

Section 19.1: GENITOURINARY SYSTEMS

The urinary system is composed of the two kidneys, two ureters, the bladder, adrenals, and the urethra. The purpose of the urinary system is to produce, store, and eliminate urine. The kidneys are designated by the combining forms nephro and renal.   The kidneys' main role is to filter waste products from the blood including urea which secretes rennin, a hormone involved in the control of blood pressure which is why hypertension and chronic kidney disease are always related. The glomerulus are contained within the kidneys and part of the filtration system of the kidneys. The ureters carry urine from the kidneys to the urinary bladder. The adrenals are positioned on top of the kidneys, but they are part of the endocrine system.

Testes are contained within the scrotum. The sperm is produced within the seminiferous tubules which are located within the testes. The perineum is located between the scrotum and the anus. The prostate gland lies where the vas deferens meets the urethra.

The female genital organs include the uterus and the ovaries which are located in the pelvis above the uterus and connected to the uterus through the fallopian tubes. The lower narrow portion of the uterus is the cervix. The vagina extends downward from the uterus to an orifice to the exterior of the body. The perineum is the area between the orifice and the anus. This is the area that may be cut (episiotomy) during delivery to prevent tearing.

Adnexa is sometimes used to refer to appendages of an organ which are anatomical parts attached to that organ. For example, the ovaries and oviducts are the adnexa uteri as they are considered part of the uterus since they are attached.

Section 19.2: GLOMERULAR DISEASES

Glomerular disease (N00-N08) does not include hypertensive kidney failure which is coded as N17-N19. It does include nephritic and nephrotic syndromes (N00-N05) which can be acute, rapidly progressive or recurrent/persistent. It can include various associated glomerulonephritis as described in the specific codes. Glomerulonephritis is inflammation of the glomeruli (small blood vessels in the kidneys). Proliferative indicates that there is an increased number of cells in the glomerulus and this usually leads to end-stage renal disease (ESRD) and failure (ESRF).

Nephrotic syndrome is a condition that results from another condition, such as diabetes, in which the kidneys are damaged, causing them to leak large amounts of protein from the blood into the urine. This condition is demonstrated by labs that indicate proteinuria, hyperlipidemia, edema, and hypoalbuminemia. These codes are also differentiated by the presence of lesions and proliferation.

Recurrent and persistent hematuria is coded as N02. Proteinuria is coded as N06 with various associated conditions such as glomerular lesions and glomerulonephritis. Hereditary nephropathy is coded as N07. Glomerular disorders can occur in diseases (N08) such as amyloidosis, congenital syphilis, gout, sepsis, and sickle cell.

Renal tubule-interstitial disease (N10-N16) include nephritis of these anatomic sites such as pyelonephritis which can be obstructive or not. Pyelonephritis (N10) (also known as pyelitis) is a suppurative infection of the kidney and can be coded as acute and/or chronic and with or without necrosis. It can be coded in various other sections as well depending upon complications and comorbidities.

Uropathy (N13) can also be obstructive such as calculus. This includes hydronephrosis and hydroureter. Strictures or kinking (N13.5) are narrowing of the urethra which may result in incontinence (involuntary leakage of urine) and are differentiated by cause, such as inflammation or scarring. Vesicoureteral reflux is the backflow of urine from the bladder into the ureter which is differentiated as being either unilateral or bilateral and with or without nephropathy.

Other diseases can result from drug and heavy metal exposure (N14) and other diseases (N16) such as brucellosis and leukemia.

Section 19.3: RENAL FAILURE/DISEASE

Renal failure is coded as N17 for acute and N18 for chronic. If the condition is hypertensive renal disease, then it is coded as I12.0 and if there is heart disease involved, then code I13 would be used, not the N codes.

While there is much emphasis on chronic renal failure, renal failure can be acute due to necrosis, lesions, toxins, shock, or injury although acute renal failure due to traumatic injury would be coded as T56.3X1A. The underlying condition should also be coded. Hyperkalemia can occur from this which is elevated potassium in the blood which can result in muscles weakness and cardiac arrest.

Chronic Kidney Disease (CKD) is a gradual progressive loss of renal function that results in end stage renal disease (ESRD). Hemodialysis or peritoneal dialysis are used to help control the effects of chronic kidney disease.

Chronic kidney diseases are classified by stages, ranging from I to V with an additional code for end-stage renal disease (ESRD) (N18.6) and unspecified stage (N18.9). Stage II is mild, Stage III is moderate, Stage IV is severe, and Stage V is the stage before ESRD. If a patient is described as having ESRD and CKD, then only the ESRD needs to be coded.

Be sure to check the notations for this code which include a reminder that hypertension must be coded as part of the code. In addition, there is a note that a code should be listed also to indicate if the patient had a kidney transplant. Another note also directs you to code also the manifestation such as neuropathy or pericarditis.

Section 19.4: UROLITHIASIS

There are new codes for urolithiasis (N20-N23) that specify the site of the calculus.

Calculi (N20) can also occur in the urinary tract organs with common occurrences in the renal pelvis or calyces of the kidneys and are known as nephrolithiasis. These codes are differentiated by anatomic site. If these calculi become placed so they obstruct the flow of urine, this is known as hydronephrosis (N13.1) which can lead to atrophy of the kidney. A calculus can become so large that its fills the pelvis of the kidney completely and blocks the flow of urine which is known as a staghorn calculus and has to be removed surgically. Calculi can also occur in diverticulum of the bladder (N21.0) or in other areas of the lower urinary tract.

Section 19.5: OTHER DISEASES OF URINARY SYSTEM

Other disorders of kidney and ureter (N25-N29) include renal osteodystrophy, diabetes insipidus, secondary hyperparathyroidism of renal origin, contracted kidney, small kidney, ischemia and infarction of kidney, and pyelitis cystica. Renal insufficiency (N28.9) is an early stage of renal impairment when the kidneys cannot function properly or adequately.

Other diseases of the urinary system (N30-N39) include cystitis which is inflammation of the urinary bladder and ureters, oftentimes due to a vaginal infection. Cystitis is classified as interstitial, chronic, trigonitis, or irradiation. Cystitis may also occur with the formation of cysts which is known as cystitis cystica.

There are a wide variety of conditions that can occur with the urinary bladder (N32), including fistulas, obstruction, atony (loss of muscle strength), overactivity, diverticulum, neurogenic (dysfunction in the micturition (voiding) due to diseases of the central nervous system or peripheral nerves) such as flaccid, reflex or uninhibited. If urinary incontinence is present, it should also be coded (N39.4).

Urethritis (N34) is inflammation of the urethra and can be with abscesses, nongonococcal or postmenopausal. Urethral strictures (N35) can be post-traumatic or postinfective. Other disorders of the urethra (N36) include fistulas, diverticulum, caruncle, functional and muscular disorders, false passage and involved in other disease.

Urinary tract infections not otherwise specified (NOS) are coded as N39.0. Additional codes should be listed to identify the infectious organism. Included in this section is stress incontinence which requires that any associated overactive bladder also be coded with N32 codes. Other incontinence includes urge incontinence, post-void dribbling, nocturnal enuresis, continuous leakage and mixed.

Section 19.6: DISEASES OF MALE GENITAL ORGANS

Diseases of male genital organs (N40-N53) include enlarged prostate (N40), better known as benign prostatic hyperplasia (BPH) as well as other similar conditions. BPH is the enlargement of the prostate in men, but this is a misnomer because the enlargement is due to hyperplasia rather than hypertrophy. These codes can include lower urinary tract syndrome and can be either nodular or enlarged. Associated symptoms should also be coded such as nocturia or straining on urination.

These codes do not include neoplasms of the prostate which are coded with neoplasm codes, such as C61.

Prostatitis (N41) is inflammation of the prostate which can be acute, chronic or with an abscess or cyst. If an organism is known to have caused the prostatitis, then the organism should be coded first. Other disorders of the prostate include calculus, congestion, hemorrhage, dysplasia, and cysts.

Hydrocele and spermatocele (N43) are accumulations of fluid in any cavity or duct. They can be encysted or infected. Noninflammatory disorders of testis (N44) include torsion (twisted) and cysts. Orchitis and epididymitis (N45) are inflammation of the testis or epididymis.

Male infertility (N46) includes azoospermia (lack of sperm), oligospermia (reduced number of sperm), or other causes such as drugs, infection, or obstruction.

Disorders of the prepuce (N47) include phimosis (tightness of the foreskin), deficient foreskin, cysts, adhesions, and inflammation.

Disorders of the penis (N48) include balanitis which is inflammation of the penis, leukoplakia, priapism (painful erection), ulcers, and induration. The underlying cause should be coded. Inflammatory disorders (N49) include Fournier gangrene, abscesses, boils, and cellulitis.

Male erectile dysfunction (N52) can be vasculogenic, drug-induced, post-surgical, or other. Other sexual dysfunctions include ejaculatory dysfunction (N53.1) such as retarded, painful and retrograde.

Section 19.7: BREASTS DISORDERS

This section is small but has conditions that apply to men and women. TheN60-N65 codes refer to dysplasias of the female mammaries. This includes cysts, fibroadenosis, and fibrosclerosis.

Other disorders include inflammatory disease, hypertrophy, galactorrhea (inappropriate discharge of milk), mastodynia (pain in the breasts), lumps (not cancerous), and ptosis (drooping of breasts). Hypertrophy of breasts (N62) include gynecomastia which is the development of breasts in men.

Section 19.8: GYNECOLOGIC DISORDERS

There are a wide variety of inflammatory diseases (N70-N77) of the various anatomic sites. Sometimes one code may contain several anatomic sites, such as salpingitis and oophoritis which are coded as N70 and can also include oophoritis. These codes can also be used for abscesses, pyosalpinx and tubo-ovarian inflammatory disease.

Inflammation of the uterus (N71) includes pyometra and endometritis. Cervicitis (N72) is inflammation of the cervix which can be acute and/or chronic. Vaginitis is inflammation of the vagina.

Other female pelvic inflammatory diseases (N73) include parametritis and pelvic cellulitis, peritonitis, and peritoneal adhesions. Peritoneal adhesions are internal scar tissue that forms after infection. If the adhesions are due to surgery then it should be coded as N99.4. This can result in infertility.

Pelvic inflammatory disease PID NOS is coded as N73.9. PID in disorders in other diseases is coded as N74. Cysts, abscesses or other diseases of Bartholin's gland are coded as N75. Vaginitis, ulcers, and abscesses of the vagina and vulva are coded as N76.

Noninflammatory disorders (N80-N98) include endometriosis which occurs when endometrial tissue is located outside of the lining of the uterine cavity which can result in painful menstruation (dysmenorrhea). Codes are differentiated by anatomic sites.

Genital prolapse (N81) is the collapse of the uterus and/or vagina from its normal position so that it falls or sinks. It can be incomplete or complete. Prolapse codes are differentiated by the presence of a cele. A cystocele is a herniation in which the bladder enters into the vagina. Urethrocele is when the urethra prolapses into the vagina. Rectocele is a hernia in which there is a tear that allows the rectal tissue to bulge through this tear into the vagina. Cystoceles/cystourethroceles can be midline or lateral.

Fistulas (N82) are differentiated by anatomic sites. Other disorders include cysts (N83), atrophy, torsion of ovaries and fallopian tubes, hematomas, polyps (N84), endometrial hyperplasia (N85), hypertrophy, inversion, or malposition of the uterus. Cervical dysplasia (N87) is the abnormal growth of cells in the cervix which can be a precursory sign of cancer and can be mild or moderate.

Other noninflammatory disorders of the cervix (N88) include leukoplakia, old laceration, stricture, stenosis, incompetence and hypertrophic elongation of the cervix. Other noninflammatory disorders of the vagina (N89) include dysplasia (mild or moderate), dysplasia, leukoplakia, tight hymenal ring or hematocolpos. N90 codes are similar to N88 and N89 codes but are for the vulva and perineum. These also include codes for female genital mutilation, Type 1 to Type IV status.

Absent, scanty, or rare menstruation (N91) can be primary or secondary amenorrhea or oligomenorrhea. Excessive, frequent or irregular (N92) menstruation can occur at different times such as premenopausal or at puberty. Metrorrhagia is bleeding in between menstruation periods.

Dyspareunia (painful sexual intercourse) and primary or secondary dysmenorrhea are coded as N94. Dysmenorrhea is painful menstruation. Menopausal and climacteric states (N95) include flushing, sleeplessness, headache, and lack of concentration. The associated symptoms should also be coded.

If a woman has continued to have miscarriages from (three or more consecutive) pregnancies at approximately the same time, usually before 20 weeks of gestation, then this is known as an habitual aborter (N96); however, if she is pregnant, then O26 should be used as the code instead.

Infertility issues (N97) include the cause, such as lack of ovulation, endocrine complications, and anatomic site of problem. Complications associated with artificial fertilization (N98) include infection, hyperstimulation of ovaries, and various complications.

Intraoperative and postprocedural complications or genitourinary system (N99) include kidney failure, urethral stricture, adhesions, prolapse, complications of stoma of the urinary tract (hemorrhage, infection, and malfunction), hemorrhage, hematoma, accidental puncture or laceration, and others.

GENITOURINARY QUIZ 13

1. What are the codes for a patient with acute pyelonephritis due to E. coli?

2. What are the codes for a patient with oophoritis and salpingitis?

3. What are the codes for a patient with chronic uremia with acute pericarditis?

4. What are the codes for a patient with urinary incontinence and genital prolapse?

5. What are the codes for a patient with orchitis and epididymitis due to diphtheria?

6. What are the codes for a patient with menorrhagia?

7. What are the codes for a patient with post-hysterectomy vaginal prolapse?

8. What are the codes for a patient with acute cholecystitis with bile duct calculus with obstruction?

9. What are the codes for a patient with subacute nonsuppurative nephritis?

10. What are the codes for a patient with renal disease with membranous proliferative glomerulonephritis?

11. What are the codes for a patient with diverticulitis of the ileum with hemorrhage and peritonitis?

12. What are the codes for a patient with vesicoureteral reflux with bilateral reflux nephropathy?

13. What are the codes for a patient with ureteral calculus and renal calculus?

14. What are the codes for a patient with posttraumatic renal failure?

15. What are the codes for a patient with septic UTI due to E. coli?

CHAPTER 20
ICD-10 PREGNANCY

You will learn the following objectives in this chapter:

A. Pregnancy Definitions
    1. Gynecology/Obstetrics
    2. Fertilization
    3. Antepartum
    4. Delivery
B. Indentations
C. Coding Scenarios
    1. Unrelated Condition
    2. Related Condition as Combination Code
    3. Related Condition as Multiple Codes
D. Abortions
    1. Spontaneous
    2. Induced
    3. Ectopic Pregnancies
    4. Molar Pregnancies
E. High Risk Pregnancies
F. Eclampsia
G. Gestational
H. Other Disorders During Pregnancy
I. Multiple Gestations
J. Maternal Care for Other Complications
    1. Malpresentations
    2. Disproportions
K. Placental Conditions
L. Delivery
    1. Outcome of Birth
M. Complications
N. Postpartum
O. Infections
P. Other Conditions
Q. Sterilizations

Chapter 15 is described as "Pregnancy, Childbirth and the Puerperium" and ranges from O00-O9A. Be careful when using these codes because the use of the alphabetical O should not be confused with the number zero.

Section 20.1: GYNECOLOGY/OBSTETRICS

Gynecology is the study of female reproduction and obstetrics. Obstetrics is the study of pregnancy. Neonatology is the study of newborns and will not be covered in this packet because neonates have their own ICD-10 codes; only the mother should be coded from obstetric codes.

The gonads of the male and female produce gametes. The female gonads are the ovaries and the male gonads are the testes. The female gamete is the ovum and the male is the sperm.

When the ovum and a sperm cell unite, then fertilization has occurred and the fertilized ovum is known as an embryo. After two months, it is known as a fetus.

The embryo is fed through the placenta that grows in the wall of the uterus throughout the pregnancy. The unborn child grows within the amnion cavity, which is filled with fluid which is known as the sack of water. As you may remember from our discussion about blood, the mother's and baby's blood never mix.

The hormones, estrogen and progesterone, provide major control over the course of the pregnancy. The placenta also produces a hormone, human chorionic gondadotropin (HCG) whose presence indicates pregnancy.

A pregnancy is also known as gestation. It usually lasts 40 weeks (9 months). Dates are very important to know when coding pregnancy and delivery conditions.

Gravidity (G) refers to the number of pregnancies. Parity (P) refers to the number of viable pregnancies (approximately viable at 22 weeks). With these terms, a woman may be classified as G2 P1 Ab1 which means two pregnancies, one viable pregnancy, and one abortion.

Antepartum is the period preceding the delivery which is usually 40 weeks.

Delivery is the birth of the baby. The expulsion of the placenta is also known as the afterbirth. Delivery is also known as parturition.

Postpartum is also known as puerperium which refers to time beginning immediately after delivery and extending until six weeks following delivery. However, puerperium's true definition is the time required for the uterus to return to its normal size.

Section 20.2: INDENTATIONS

This is one of the most difficult sections to code from in the alphabetical index, similar to neoplasms, because there are so many categories, alternate terms, subterms, and indentations which make it extremely easy to select a wrong code from the wrong terms. As discussed in earlier packets, you must follow the alphabetical order of the sections, particularly since some alternate terms have very long sections within the pregnancy codes, such as "due to", "management affected by", "complicated by", etc. However, perhaps one of the greatest attributes of the ICD10 book is that it uses grey bars in the alphabetical index which indicate indentations so that it is much easier to know if a description is included under a section or if it is under a different section.

In addition, if you do not find a condition listed, it may still be listed in the pregnancy codes but under its own or alternate terms, so be sure to check all of these terms before you decide if the condition is not listed under the pregnancy codes. If you do find the condition under its own or alternate terms then use that code as it will cross-reference to any other descriptions. For example, vomiting in a pregnant patient is selected from the alphabetical index under the terms "complicated by" within the pregnancy codes.

Section 20.3: CODING SCENARIOS

When a patient is pregnant, for any condition a coder should begin searching under the terms pregnancy, delivery, or labor depending upon the stage of the pregnancy for that condition. There are several coding scenarios that can occur:

UNRELATED CONDITION: The first scenario for coding when a patient is pregnant is demonstrated in the fracture scenario. Since fracture is not listed under the term "pregnancy", then the fracture should be coded in addition to Z33.1 (incidental pregnancy).

RELATED CONDITION AS COMBINATION CODE: For the second scenario, as demonstrated in the UTI scenario, the coding becomes more complicated. If a condition is found under pregnancy, such as excessive vomiting, then the pregnancy code with the condition should be listed (O21). These codes include both the pregnancy and the condition and does not have any notations requiring the use of another code, so this one code includes both.

RELATED CONDITION AS MULTIPLE CODES: For the third scenario, if, and only if, there is a notation in the tabular index under the code that says another code must also be listed, such as another condition, then additional codes must be listed. For example superficial thrombophlebitis in pregnancy would be coded as O22.2 which requires the additional coding of the thrombophlebitis as I80.0.

Section 20.4: ABORTIONS

Abortion is defined as the termination of a pregnancy by the expulsion of the fetus. Abortions are natural (spontaneous) or induced (legally or illegally).

Ectopic pregnancy is when the embryo implants in a site other than the uterus. Most of these occur within the fallopian tubes and, therefore, are also known as tubal pregnancies. Other sites for ectopic pregnancies include the ovaries and other specified sites. Ectopic pregnancies are coded as O00 with a fourth character for the site.

Molar pregnancies (O02) are an abnormal growth in pregnancy in which a hydatidiform mole is formed from the fertilization of the egg and sperm but no viable fetus is formed due to a lack of the nucleus in the egg. They are also known as gestational trophoblastic disease (GTD).

Other types of abnormal conception products include blighted ovum, molar pregnancy, missed abortions and inappropriate change in HCG during pregnancy. Associated complications should be coded additionally with codes O08.

If complications occurs from these types of pregnancies or abortions, such as septic shock, sepsis, hemorrhage, damage to organs, renal failure, or embolism, then these should be coded from the O08.0 codes.

A missed abortion (O02.1) occurs when fetus dies before 20 weeks gestation in utero but this was not known and the fetus remained in the uterus. If this occurred after 22 weeks, then it is coded as O36.4. If the fetus remains in the uterus for more than 6 weeks it is known as dead fetus syndrome and it is included in the O02.1 and O36.4 codes.

Codes O03 are for the type of abortion, spontaneous, medical, or other. The fourth character indicates if the abortion was complete or incomplete and if there are any complications.

In a spontaneous abortions (O03) the codes are differentiated as to whether they are complete or incomplete and by associated complications and conditions such as genital tract or pelvic infection, hemorrhage, embolism, shock, renal failure, metabolic disorder, damage to pelvic organs, sepsis, and cardiac arrest. Incomplete means some products of the pregnancy are retained in the uterus after the abortion.

If a woman has continued to have miscarriages from (three or more consecutive) pregnancies at approximately the same time, usually before 20 weeks of gestation, then she should be coded as a habitual (recurrent) aborter (N96). However, if she is pregnant and it has not resulted in an abortion, then O26.2 should be used as the code instead. It is important to code this condition because it does present a high risk for the mother. In addition, a code for a history of abortions can be listed (O09.29).

An induced abortion can occur at any time including up until the birth of the baby as long as a portion of the baby remains within the mother. If an abortion fails, then it would be coded as O07. A therapeutic abortion is performed for reasons related to the health of the mother. An elective abortion occurs for other reasons. These codes are differentiated by associated complications and conditions such as infection, hemorrhage, embolism, shock, renal failure, metabolic disorder, damage to organs, cardiac arrest, and sepsis.

If an abortion is performed to reduce the number of fetuses, then it is coded as O31. There is also a code for Encounter for elective termination of pregnancy, Z33.2, which should also be coded when patient presents for an induced abortion. A failed attempted abortion would be coded as O07. Incomplete abortions are not considered failed and should not be coded with these codes. Codes O04 are used when there are complications from the abortion, e.g. termination of pregnancy complicated by embolism (O04.7). Complications following ectopic and molar pregnancies are coded as O08, e.g. shock following ectopic and molar pregnancy (O08.3).

Section 20.5: HIGH-RISK PREGNANCY

Supervision of high-risk pregnancies (O09) now require the specification of history in the fourth character and trimester in the fifth. History can include infertility, ectopic/molar pregnancy, poor past reproductive events, multiparity, elderly gravida, young gravida, and social problems.

Multiparity indicates that mother is or has had deliveries in the past in which more than one baby was born which definitely constitutes high risk. If the mother is expecting multiple births, then O09.4 should be listed in addition to any other pregnancy codes. However, if the mother had presented for delivery then O30 codes can be used to indicate the multiplicity. If a mother has a history of multiple births, then code Z64.1 can be coded as it provides important information about the possibility of future multiple births which are high-risk pregnancies.

If a pregnant woman is 35 years or older for her first pregnancy, then that would be coded as elderly primigravida (O09.51). If this is not her first pregnancy, then the code for elderly multigravida (O09.52) would be used. If a pregnant woman is less than 16 years of age, then it would be coded as O09.6-.

A mother may undergo fetal reduction (O31.3) to reduce the number of fetuses when there is a multiple birth, such as reduction in which one of twins may be terminated while the other twin remains viable.

Section 20.6: ECLAMPSIA

Conditions related to eclampsia are coded as O10-O16. Preeclampsia is pregnancy-induced hypertension and toxemia as indicated by high blood pressure, excessive protein in the urine (proteinuria), and edema. Eclampsia is characterized by tonic-clonic seizures in a patient who had pre-eclampsia. This is a very dangerous condition which is why these conditions are tested regularly during pregnancy.

Eclampsia is preceded by pre-eclampsia which is diagnosed by the presence of hypertension (with heart disease or kidney disease), proteinuria, and edema either alone or in combination (O10-O16) but not all three (which is coded as eclampsia.) Further specification for M10 includes a fourth character for nature of the hypertension, fifth character indicating if the hypertension is affecting the pregnancy, and a sixth character for the trimester involved, e.g. pre-existing hypertensive heart disease complicating pregnancy, second trimester (O10.112).

Section 20.7: GESTATIONAL

Conditions may arise during pregnancy that did not exist when the woman was not pregnant. This includes gestational (transient) high blood pressure (O13) and gestational diabetes (O24) which will disappear after the pregnancy is completed.

Section 20.8: OTHER DISORDERS DURING PREGNANCY

Other disorders that can occur during pregnancy include hemorrhage and vomiting. If vomiting occurs, the code is selected based on when the vomiting began and complications. If it began before the end of 20 weeks' gestation, then it is coded as mild hyperemesis gravidarum (O21.0). If it began before 20 weeks' gestation and involved dehydration, electrolyte disturbance, or carbohydrate depletion, then it is coded as O21.1. If the vomiting began after 20 weeks' gestation, then it is coded as O21.2.

A threatened abortion (O20.0) occurs when there is bleeding before 20 weeks without expulsion of the fetus and without dilation of the cervix. Hemorrhage is coded as O20.

Venous complications (O22) include hemorrhoids, varicose veins, genital varices, thrombophlebitis (superficial or deep), and thrombosis.

Infections during pregnancy (O23) can occur in the kidneys, bladder, urethra and other anatomic sites. The fifth character indicates the trimester when the infection occurs.

Diabetic codes (O24) during pregnancy have also been expanded with the fourth character indicating if the diabetes is pre-existing or gestational. The fifth character indicates when the gestation occurs such as in pregnancy, in childbirth or in the puerperium. The sixth characters indicated trimester involved and if the diabetes is controlled.

Diet and weight conditions affecting pregnancy (O25-O26) include malnutrition and excessive or low weight gain as well as recurrent pregnancy loss and retained intrauterine contraceptive device during pregnancy.

Other conditions (O26) include herpes during the pregnancy, hypotension, liver/biliary tract disorders, subluxation of pubis bone, exhaustion, fatigue, neuritis, renal disease, size-date discrepancy of the pregnancy, spotting, and cervical shortening.

Section 20.9: MULTIPLE GESTATIONS

Multiple gestations (O30) include twin, triplet, quadruplet or other. The fifth characters indicate further define the multiplicity such as if the twins are conjoined, number of placenta and amniotic sacs. Complications due to multiplicity (O31) include papyraceous fetus, pregnancy that continued after spontaneous abortion or death or reduction of one of the fetuses. Seventh characters indicate how many fetus there are. Papyraceous fetus is known as the "vanishing" twin as it is being compressed by the other fetus and dies.

Section 20.10: MATERNAL CARE FOR OTHER COMPLICATIONS

There are various conditions (O32-O47) that require additional maternal care beyond that provided for a normal pregnancy which may require additional observation, hospitalization, or other obstetric care as well as possible cesarean section. . These include malpresentations. Malpresentations (O32) occurs when the baby does not present head first. These include breech, unstable lie, transverse/oblique, face/brow/chin, high head, compound, and footling. A breech birth occurs when the baby's head does not present first but instead the feet do; if one foot is presented first this is known as footling. Usually with malpresentations, the doctor will attempt to correct it by manual manipulation to turn the baby around before delivery. There are other codes to use if the malpresentation complicates delivery with codes O64.

Disproportion (O33) includes problems such as deformity of the mother's pelvic bones, contracted pelvis, outlet contraction, or disproportion between mother and babies. A seventh character indicates how many babies are involved during this pregnancy. Different codes are used if disproportion presents during the delivery with codes O64 codes.

Other conditions include congenital malformations of the mother's uterus, tumors, and scar from previous C-section. Abnormalities of the pregnant uterus can include incarceration, prolapse, and retroversion. There are also abnormalities that occur in the vagina, vulva and perineum. These codes are differentiated by the trimester involved. An incarcerated uterus is trapped in the pelvis. Retroversion is when the uterus has tipped backwards.

Fetal conditions can affect the outcome of the pregnancy as well as the mother's health; therefore, there are pregnancy codes (O35) provided for these conditions but they are codes for the effect or possible effect on the mother, not the fetus. These may include genetic malformations of the baby, damage to the baby, decreased fetal movements, and fetal distress.

Isoimmunizations occurs when there is possible incompatibility between mother and baby which includes the Rh factor (O36) and blood types. Intrauterine death of the baby is coded as O36.4.

Fetal conditions also include if the baby is large or small. If a baby is small, it is known as "light for dates" and is coded as poor fetal growth (O36.5). If the baby is large, it is known as "large for dates" and is coded as excessive fetal growth (O36.6). These conditions must be described by the physician and should not be determined by the coder.

Section 20.11: PLACENTAL CONDITIONS

Various conditions of the amniotic sac and membranes can provide complications (O41-O45). This includes infections and premature rupture of the membranes (water sac breaking) with onset of labor within or after 24 hours after and if this occurs prematurely or preterm. Preterm occurs before 37 weeks gestation. These code are differentiated by trimester involved.

Placental disorders (O43) include transfusion syndrome that can involve the transfer between mother and baby or between babies if multiple births. Other disorders of the placenta include malformation, circumvallate, velamentous insertion of umbilical cord, placenta accrete, placenta increta, placenta percreta, and infarction. Placenta accrete is when the placenta is too deeply and firmly attached in the uterus. Placenta increta is when the placenta attaches in the muscular wall of the uterus. Placenta percreta is when the placenta grows through the uterus.

Placenta previa (O44) is when the placenta is implanted at the lower end of the uterus which can result in a lack of adequate oxygen. These code are differentiated as to with or without hemorrhage.

Abruptio placentae (O45) is when the placenta separates prematurely from the wall and is an emergency. These codes are differentiated by the presence of various conditions such as coagulation defect. Trimester is coded with the sixth character.

Antepartum hemorrhage (O46) is coded with the inclusion of various complications including coagulation defect, afibrinogenemia, or disseminated intravascular coagulation.

Section 20.12: DELIVERY

Gestational age at delivery should be coded additionally if it is not normal (normal is between 37 to 40 weeks). Preterm refers to deliveries prior to 38 weeks gestation and so there should be an additional code listed for early onset (O60) as it does present risks. A pregnancy that ends before 37 weeks of gestation resulting in a live-born infant is known as a premature birth. Preterm labor is threatened labor during this time period which does not result in delivery.

False labor (O47) is known as Braxton Hicks contraction or threated labor. Codes are differentiated as occurring before 37 completed weeks or after and as being in either the second or third trimester. False labor (O47) codes are differentiated by completed weeks of gestation and trimester, either before or after 37 weeks.

Term refers to deliveries between 38 and 40 weeks and do not require any additional codes.

Postterm refers to deliveries between 40 and 42 weeks which are coded as late pregnancies (O48.0) and prolonged is after 42 weeks.

Various conditions can affect delivery. This includes multiple gestations which are coded as O30-O31 and complications due to multiple gestation are coded as O31. Malpresentation of fetus is coded as O32. Vaginal delivery following a previous C-section is coded as O75.7. Single delivery is coded as O80. C-section is coded as O82 if not performed due to any complications; otherwise it is included with the complication precipitating its use. Outcome of delivery is coded as Z37.

Codes for complications of anesthesia during pregnancy have been expanded to include complications during pregnancy (O29), during delivery (O74) and during the puerperium (O89). The complication and trimester are further specified by the fourth and fifth characters. Complications can include aspiration pneumonitis, lung collapse, cardiac arrest or failure, cerebral anoxia, toxic reaction, headache, and failed or difficult intubation.

If induction of delivery is attempted but fails, then it would be coded as O61 and are defined as medical, instrumental, or other. If labor is attempted by fails to deliver this is coded as O66.4 which includes failed attempted VBAC (vaginal birth after previous C-section). If vacuum extractor or forceps are used code O66.5 should be used even if the delivery still occurs with the use of the forceps or by C-section.

Abnormalities of labor forces (O62) include inadequate, arrested, hypotonic, atony, irregular labor, and poor contractions. Labor that is fast is known as precipitate. Prolonged contractions are coded as O62.4. If the labor is prolonged (more than 24 hours) then it would be coded with O63 codes as determined by stages of labor, either first, second, delayed or long.

A normal delivery with the birth of a live born is coded as O82 with no other characters required. If anything else occurs other than an episiotomy, then it is not considered a normal delivery and should be coded from other pregnancy codes that describe other conditions or problems existed.

Cesarean delivery is coded under the complication code such as for disproportion or atony. These can all be found in the alphabetical index under delivery, cesarean. Cesarean delivery occurs when the baby is delivered surgically through the abdomen rather than vaginally. The C-section itself is a procedure and would be coded with the CPT codes.

If a woman delivers, whether it is vaginal or Cesarean (C-section), but had a C-section before, this should be noted with the use of code O34.21. If she has a vaginal birth, but had a C-section before, this is known as VBAC, vaginal birth after Cesarean. The woman may have a vaginal or Cesarean delivery after having had a previous Cesarean section, but this can pose some risks.

OUTCOMES OF BIRTH: When the visit is for delivery, then a code must be listed for the outcome of the births using Z37 codes. A single live born is coded as Z37.0 which constitutes most deliveries. Z37.1 is a single stillborn birth, Z37.2 is for live born twins, Z37.3 is for one live born and one stillborn twins and these classifications culminate in Z37.9 which is for unknown outcome. When a fetus dies in utero after about 20 weeks, or during delivery, it is usually termed stillborn.

Section 20.13: COMPLICATIONS

As described earlier, other than a normal delivery, all other complications must be coded with pregnancy codes other than O80. Complications include medical conditions but can also include labor and delivery issues, such as obstructed labor (O64) or trauma to the perineum or vulva of the mother (O71). Obstructed labor can occur due to the size of the baby, size of mother's pelvis, or other complication. Obstructed labor due to malposition or malpresentations of the baby use codes O64. Physical conditions of the mother's pelvis that complicate delivery are coded as O65 such as deformed or contracted pelvis.

Labor or delivery complicated by hemorrhage is coded as O67. Postpartum hemorrhages (O72) include third-stage hemorrhage with retained placenta, immediate, secondary, delayed, or postpartum coagulation defects.

Various complications with the umbilical cord can complicate delivery (O69). These include prolapse of the cord, cord around the neck of the baby with compression, other types of cord entanglements, short cord, and various conditions of the cord such as hemorrhage, hematoma, bruising, and thrombosis.

If the perineum is lacerated during delivery this is coded as O70. It is differentiated as first, second, third, or fourth degree. There is also a code if the sphincter is torn. Similar complications include rupture of the uterus (O71) either before or during labor, inversion of the uterus, obstetric laceration of the uterus, or hematoma of the pelvis.

Other complications of labor and delivery (O75) include maternal distress, shock, pyrexia, infections, cardiac arrest or failure, cerebral anoxia, maternal exhaustion, and pulmonary edema. If there are abnormalities in the baby's heart rate and rhythm during labor and delivery this is coded as O76 which can include bradycardia (slow), tachycardia (fast), irregularity, or deceleration. Fetal distress is coded as O77.

Section 20.14: POSTPARTUM/PUERPERUM

Complications encountered after labor and delivery (O85-O92) include sepsis and other infections such as cervicitis, vaginitis, pyrexia, and urinary tract infection. Venous complications include thrombophlebitis, hemorrhoids, thrombosis, or embolisms. Embolism can be air, amniotic fluid, pyemic, septic, or thromboembolism. Complications from anesthesia are coded as O89 which includes cardiac or CNS complications or failed intubation. Other complications include disruption/dehiscence of surgical repair such as C-section, hematoma, cardiomyopathy, kidney failure, thyroiditis, and mood disturbance (postpartum blues or dysphoria).

Infections of the breast associated with pregnancy (O91) include infections of the nipples, abscesses, mastitis, retracted nipples, cracked nipples, aglactia, and suppressed lactation.

Sequelae of complications of pregnancy, childbirth and puerperium are coded as O94. The actual condition should be coded first.

Section 20.15: INFECTIONS

Infections or parasitic diseases (O98) complicating pregnancy, childbirth or puerperium include tuberculosis, syphilis, gonorrhea, viral hepatitis, protozoal, and HIV. The organism should also be coded if known.

Section 20.16: OTHER CONDITIONS

Other conditions complicating the pregnancy, childbirth or puerperium (O99) include anemia, other blood problems, obesity, endocrine conditions, mental including alcohol or drug abuse, circulatory and pulmonary conditions, as well as liver and skin. Other conditions also include abnormal glucose levels, Step B carrier, bariatric surgery, malignant neoplasm, injury, poisoning, and physical, sexual or psychological abuse. O9A is for neoplasms, injury, poisonings, and all types of abuse.

Section 20.17: STERILIZATION

Sterilization codes are not coded from either the genitourinary or pregnancy codes, so they will be discussed in a later packet. However, if the reason for the sterilization is either genitourinary or pregnancy, then those codes would be selected from these chapters.

PREGNANCY QUIZ 14

1) What are the codes for a 36-year-old pregnant woman who has a C section due to fetal distress at 39 weeks?

2) What are the codes for a 25-year-old pregnant woman who is 33-weeks gestation, has gestational diabetes and is seen today for dehydration?

3) What are the codes for an 18-year-old pregnant woman who has difficulty in labor due to the birth of a 12 pound baby boy?

4) What are the codes for a pregnant woman who delivered liveborn twins with one normal and the other breech at 32 weeks with both weighing 5 pounds?

5) What are the codes for a pregnant woman who has had three previous miscarriages at approximately 18 weeks and presents today at 20 weeks gestation who is experiencing cramping?

6) What are the codes for a 39-year-old pregnant woman whose baby at 32-weeks gestation is known to have Down's syndrome?

7) What are the codes for a pregnant 23-year-old woman who delivered by C-section a liveborn today at 35 weeks due to severe eclampsia and decreased fetal movement?

8) What are the codes for a pregnant woman who delivered a liveborn girl which required an episiotomy to aid in delivery?

9) What are the codes for a pregnant woman who delivered twins with a normal delivery?

10) What are the codes for a 25-year-old pregnant woman who delivered a 10 pound baby boy but the mother's pelvic was too small and forceps had to be used but when these did not work a C-section was done?

11) What are the codes for a 38-year-old pregnant woman, 37 weeks gestation, who is seen today for her checkup?

12) What are the codes for a pregnant 31-year-old woman who is seen today for deep thrombophlebitis which she developed four days after her delivery of liveborn at 42 weeks?

13) What are the codes for a pregnant woman who had an induced abortion two days ago and is admitted for a severe infection?

14) What are the codes for a pregnant woman who was in a car accident and fractured her tibia?

15) What are the codes for a woman who delivered a liveborn vaginally at 39 weeks and who had a C-section for her previous pregnancy?

CHAPTER 21
ICD-10 PERINATAL

You will learn the following objectives in this chapter:

A. Definitions
    1. Fetal
    2. Perinatal
    3. Newborn
    4. Neonatal
    5. Pediatric
B. Maternal Conditions
C. Malpresentations
D. Other Complications
E. Outcome of Birth
F. Fetal Growth and Malnutrition
G. Birth Trauma
H. Respiratory/Cardiovascular
I. Infections
J. Hemorrhagic
K. Endocrine/Metabolic
L. Digestive
M. Integumentary
N. Other Conditions

Chapter 16 is described as "Certain Conditions Originating in the Perinatal Period" and ranges from P00-P96. There are many new codes and expansions in these codes.

Section 21.1: DEFINITIONS

AGES: The term "fetus" is not used but rather "newborn" is used in the code descriptions. Newborn, therefore, refers to an unborn child up until the 28 days after birth.

Perinatal is the period occurring during pregnancy, specifically from 22 completed weeks of gestation to 28 completed days after birth. Although codes are listed for perinatal conditions which are defined as up until the newborn is 28 days of age, conditions that are diagnosed after this time period but were related to this time period can still be identified as perinatal. For example, if a patient suffers conditions that resulted from anoxia during birth, then associated conditions would be coded as perinatal even if they persist into later years of age.

Pediatric refers to a child who is 24 months of age or less, but older than 28 days. However, the term is also used generally to refer to a child of any age, usually up to the age of 16, but for the purposes of coding pediatric will refer to a child who is 24 months of age or less but older than 28 days.

Section 21.2: MATERNAL CONDITIONS

There may be maternal conditions that influence or affect the care of a newborn (P00). These codes are for the baby and not the mother who has her own codes for related conditions. This includes hypertension, renal and urinary tract problem, infections, nutritional problems (such as malnutrition), injury to the mother, surgical procedure on mother or other conditions.

If a mother undergoes surgery while pregnant, codes P00.7 should be used but damage from amniocentesis is coded as P02.1.

Other maternal conditions that should be coded as they may affect the outcome of care are coded as P01 codes which includes incompetent cervix, premature rupture of membranes, oligohydramnios. Incompetent cervix is when the cervix is weak and begins to open early. Oligohydramnios is inadequate amounts of amniotic fluid in the womb during pregnancy.

Ectopic pregnancies for coding for the baby is coded as P01.4. Multiparity (twins, etc) is coded as P01.5 for the baby. Maternal death is coded as P01.6.

Section 21.3: MALPRESENTATIONS

Malpresentations of the baby before labor is coded as P01.7:

- Normal - the top of the head presents first.
- Brow – the front brow portion of the head presents first.
- Face – the face presents first.
- Frank breech - the baby's bottom comes first.
- Complete breech - the baby's bottom comes first but the feet are down by the buttocks in a cross-legged position.
- Footling breech - one or both feet come first.
- Kneeling breech - the baby is in a kneeling position, with one or both legs extended at the hips and flexed at the knees.
- Compound presentation - more than one part of the baby arrives at the same time.
- Shoulder presentation – when the shoulders present first.
- Transverse – position in which the mother's and the baby's spines make a cross or a "T" shape.
- Oblique - When the baby is positioned at an angle so that the spine is off-center from the mother's.

If there are complications for the newborn during labor due to malpresentation, these are coded as P03.0 or P03.1.

Section 21.4: OTHER COMPLICATIONS

Complications of the placenta, cord and membranes (P02) include placenta previa, placental transfusion syndrome, and prolapsed cord (P02.4). Other problems with the cord include torsion of the cord, the cord wrapped about the baby's neck, knot in the cord, entanglement of the cord, short cord, and varices. If the placenta is retained after delivery without hemorrhaging it is coded as O73 for the mother.

If forceps are required, then a code for the use of forceps should also be coded (P03.2). Codes from P03 should be used to code for other assistive method, such as vacuum extraction and C-section. Precipitate delivery (fast) is coded as P03.5.

If there are complications for the baby during labor and delivery, then these should be coded as P03 such as abnormalities in the heart rate with onset before or during delivery, meconium present, and induction of labor.

Noxious substances, such as alcohol and drugs (P04) should be coded as these can greatly influence the outcome of the baby's care. This includes narcotics, hallucinogens, cocaine, and prescriptions.

Section 21.5: OUTCOME OF BIRTH: When coding for the newborn, Z38 codes must be used to indicate their birth status, such as in the hospital. This code should be listed first when this is the newborn's admission for birth.

Section 21.6: FETAL GROWTH AND MALNUTRITION

Disorders relating to the length of gestation and fetal growth are coded as P05-P08. The codes now distinguish between light for dates (P05.0) and small for gestational age (P05.1). "Light-for-dates" means the baby is underweight for their gestation age which is further classified by the presence or absence of fetal malnutrition. If the newborn is low birth weight but it is not due slow fetal growth or fetal malnutrition, then codes P07 should be used.

Extreme immaturity is coded as P07.2 for less than 28 weeks gestation and other (P07.3) for more than 28 weeks but less than 37 weeks gestation. When both birth weight and gestational age of the newborn are provided, both should be coded with birth weight sequenced first.

Extreme immaturity is when the baby weighs less than 1000 grams. Exceptionally large baby is when the baby weighs more than 4500 grams. "Large-for-dates" or "heavy-for-dates" are babies who weight plots at over 90% for gestational age.

If a baby is born later than 40 weeks of gestation that is coded as post-term infant (P08.21) and these babies are oftentimes not "large-for-dates" because the ability of the placenta to provide sufficient nutrition begins to slow. If the gestation passes 42 weeks, then this is coded as prolonged gestation. The doctor must describe these conditions in his report in order to code them.

Section 21.7: BIRTH TRAUMA

There are many new codes for birth trauma which is coded as P10-P15 and include hemorrhage and injuries to the CNS, scalp, skeleton and peripheral nervous system.

Section 21.8: RESPIRATORY/CARDIOVASCULAR

Respiratory and cardiovascular disorders in the perinatal period are coded as P19-P29. Infant respiratory distress syndrome (IRDS) (P22.0) (also known as hyaline membrane disease) is when a premature infant experiences an insufficiency of surfactant and structural immaturity of the lungs.

Birth trauma can include subdural and cerebral hemorrhage, fracture of the clavicle during delivery, and injuries to various anatomic sites such as spine and scalp.

Other respiratory conditions can include emphysema, pulmonary hemorrhage, atelectasis (when the lungs fail to fully inflate), tachypnea (rapid breathing), apnea (when breathing stops), respiratory failure, aspiration of stomach contents, respiratory arrest, and hypoxemia (absence of oxygen in blood). Various substances can be aspirated into a newborn's lungs (P23.9) that are present at the birth, including meconium, amniotic fluid, and blood.

Section 21.9: INFECTIONS

Infections related to the perinatal period are coded as P35-P39. Infections acquired before or during birth are categorized by organism or anatomic site. This includes rubella (P35.0), cytomegalovirus, herpes, candida, and tetanus. Sites include the umbilicus, breast (P37.5), and eye. If the infection spreads to sepsis/septicemia, this would also be coded as P36. If the sepsis becomes severe, it should also be coded as R65.20. Remember, the organism should also be coded.

Section 21.10: HEMORRHAGIC

Hemorrhagic and hematological disorders of the fetus and newborn are coded as P50-P61 including jaundice and Rh or blood compatibility complications.

Blood loss is coded as P50.0 for fetuses and neonates and is based on cause and/or anatomic site. If the hemorrhage or hematological disorder occurs in the newborn, then it is coded as P53.

With fetuses and neonates, if there is blood loss due to an intraventricular hemorrhage in the heart, it should be coded as P52.2 depending upon the grade. The grades depend upon where the bleeding occurs, whether in the ventricle, cerebral cortex, germinal matrix and if the ventricle is enlarged. If the hemorrhage occurs in the subarachnoid area of the head, then it is coded as P52.5. Hemorrhage of the umbilicus is coded as P51.8. Hemorrhaging evidenced by bruising, ecchymoses, hematoma, or petechiae are coded as cutaneous (P54.5).

Hemolytic disease (P55.0) is also known as erythroblastosis fetalis. It is a condition in which the red blood cells of the fetus are broken down due to the antibodies produced by the mother which were transferred to the fetus and which can result in anemia. This can result from the Rh factor, ABO blood types, and other blood grouping conflicts. Other conditions can result from this, including kernicterus (a serious form of jaundice) and hydrops fetalis (edema in the subcutaneous tissue, pleura, pericardium, or in the abdomen, also known as ascites), and these should be coded additionally, as well as late anemia.

Jaundice (icterus) is yellowish coloration to the skin due to high serum bilirubin levels caused by the breakdown of hemoglobin. Jaundice (P58.8) is coded according to cause, so the underlying condition should also be coded. This includes jaundice due to hereditary hemolytic anemia, excessive hemolysis, preterm delivery, conjugation, hepatocellular damage, and other causes. Jaundice can be conjugated or unconjugated. Unconjugated jaundice is potentially toxic and becomes conjugated when it ties itself to glucuronic acid in the liver.

Section 21.11: ENDOCRINE/METABOLIC

Endocrine and metabolic disorders (P70-P74) include infant of a diabetic mother, diabetes in the newborn, myasthenia gravis (muscle weakness and fatigue), thyrotoxicosis (abnormally high levels of thyroid hormone), hypocalcemia, hypoglycemia, and acidosis (low pH levels and bicarbonate in body fluids of neonate due to excess levels of acid).

Section 21.12: DIGESTIVE

Digestive (P76-P78) disorders in the perinatal period include obstruction by meconium (stools of unborn child), hematemesis and melena due to swallowing the mother's blood, necrotizing enterocolitis (portion of the bowels die), and perforation of the intestine.

Section 21.13: INTEGUMENTARY

Various integumentary conditions of the fetus and newborn (P80-P83) include hydrops fetalis not due to blood types, sclerema, temperature problems including hypothermia, and hydrocele. Sclerema is severe skin condition that is characterized by inflammation of the underlying subcutaneous fat.

If a baby does not obtain sufficient oxygen during delivery (P84), this can cause serious problems such as death, distress, encephalopathy, or asphyxia.

Section 21.14: OTHER CONDITIONS

Other conditions in the perinatal period include convulsions (P90), comas P91.5), feeding problems (P92) (regurgitation and slow feeding), reactions to drugs (P93), failure to thrive (P92.6), muscle tone problems (P94), renal failure (P96.8) and exposure to parental tobacco use (P96.81).

PERINATAL QUIZ 15

1) What is the code for a liveborn whose was delivered with the use of forceps at 34 weeks and weighing 1260 grams due to placentia previa?

2) What are the codes for a newborn whose mother was addicted to cocaine and the newborn is experiencing withdrawal?

3) What are the codes for a newborn at this visit who is diagnosed with neutropenia which is not transient?

4) What are the codes for a newborn with jaundice who was delivered at 34 weeks?

5) What are the codes for a 1-year-old girl who was diagnosed with sepsis due to UTI due to E. coli?

6) What are the neonatal codes for congenital TB?

7) What are the codes for a neonate who is diagnosed with diabetes?

8) What are the codes for a neonate with hyperbilirubinema who was premature at birth and so remained in the hospital with this her third day and weighed 2100 gm at birth?

9) What are the codes for a baby born at 43 weeks who experienced asphyxia due to the cord wrapped around her neck?

10) What is the code for the newborn when her mother dies during childbirth?

11) What are the codes for a patient with a bunion on the right foot?

12) What are the codes for a 1-month old baby who has not gained any weight?

13) What are the codes for a patient with lower respiratory infection?

14) What are the codes for a fetus whose mother has been diagnosed with rubella?

15) What are the codes for a newborn whose mother received an anesthetic during delivery with a C-section performed because the newborn's heart rate slowed and was in fetal distress due to the cord being wrapped about her neck with newborn suffering hypoxia?

CHAPTER 22
ICD-10 CONGENITAL

You will learn the following objectives in this chapter:

A. Congenital Conditions
    1. Acquired Versus Congenital
B. Outcome of Delivery
    1. Sequencing
    2. Congenital
C. Anomalies
    1. Cephalic
    2. Ocular
    3. Auditory
D. Congenital Heart Defects
    1. Acyanotic
    2. Cyanotic
E. Respiratory
F. Gastrointestinal/Genitourinary
    1. Cleft Lip/Palate
    2. Other GI/GU Congenital anomalies
G. Musculoskeletal
    1. Hip
    2. Legs
    3. Feet
    4. Chest
    5. Extremities
    6. Spine
    7. Bone
H. Integumentary
I. Chromosomal
J. Other Congenital Anomalies

Chapter 17 codes are for congenital malformations, deformations and chromosomal abnormalities (Q00-Q99).

Section 22.1: ACQUIRED VERSUS CONGENITAL

Acquired conditions are conditions that arise during life whereas congenital are conditions that arise during gestation and at birth and which are coded with their own codes as distinct from the acquired conditions.

Section 22.2: OUTCOME OF DELIVERY

With the mother, a Z37 code was used to designate the outcome of the birth when coding for the mother during a delivery. For the baby, delivery must be listed with Z38 codes which is always listed first. If a congenital anomaly is identified on the visit when the baby is born, then the anomaly is listed as second and the delivery is first. If the baby is transferred to another hospital or the anomaly is identified at a visit other than delivery, then only the anomaly is listed as the birth did not occur at the hospital at that time.

Section 22.3: ANOMALIES

CEPHALIC CONGENITAL ANOMALIES: Anencephalus (Q00.0) is the absence of a major portion of the brain, skull, and scalp which is due to a neural tube defect during development. Iniencephaly is when the head is bent backwards and the neck is absent due to a neural tube defect also. Encephalocele (Q01) is when a part of the cranial contents protrude through the skull. Microcephalus is a small head. Reduction deformities (Q04.3) are when part of the brain is missing or underdeveloped. Hydrocephalus (Q03.0) is when the ventricles of the brain are filled with fluid.

OCULAR CONGENITAL ANOMALIES

Congenital malformations of the eyelid, lacrimal system and orbit include ptosis, ectropion, and entropion. Ocular congenital anomalies include anophthalmos (Q11) which is the congenital absence of one or both eyes. Cryptophthalmos is when there is skin over the eyeball with absence of eyelids. Microphthalmos is when the eyes are smaller than normal. Buphthalmos is when there is increased intraocular fluid pressure which results in enlargement of the eyes. This includes congenital glaucoma (Q15.0). Cataracts (Q12.0) and other lens congenital anomalies can be congenital. Cataracts are clouding of the lens of the eye. Other congenital anomalies can involve the shape of the eye. Coloboma (Q13.0) is a hole in one of the structures of the eye. Other ocular codes include congenital anomalies of various parts of the eye, including absences and under-development.

AUDITORY CONGENITAL ANOMALIES

Congenital anomalies of the ear (Q16) can include absence of anatomic parts, hypertrophy (excessive growth), or failure to grow properly, or malformation. Atresia can occur when an anatomic site is abnormally closed or absent. There can also be fusion or development of accessory anatomic parts. Macrotia is excessive enlargement and microtia is smaller than normal sizes of part of the ear. Other deformities, such as bat ears or pointed ears are coded as Q17.5.

Section 22.4: CONGENITAL HEART DEFECTS

There are numerous congenital heart defects, some which may correct themselves with age, but others do not. These can be either cyanotic or acyanotic.

ACYANOTIC: Acyanotic means the oxygenated blood is ejected from the heart. These conditions include patent ductus arteriosis, pulmonary stenosis, atrial and ventricular septal defects, and aortic stenosis. Patent ductus arteriosis (Q25.0) is when the blood vessel connecting the ductus arteriosus (vessel connecting the aorta and the pulmonary artery) does not close shortly after birth and allows the blood to bypass the lungs. Ventricular septal defect (Q21.0) is an abnormal connection which allows the blood to pass in the wrong direction from the left ventricle to the right ventricle.

CYANOTIC: Cyanotic means there is right to left shunting of unoxygenated blood which then mixes with oxygenated blood. Common truncus (Q20.0) is a congenital anomaly in which there is abnormal connection between the ascending aorta and the pulmonary artery.

Tetralogy of Fallot (Q21.3) involves four anatomical abnormalities which are ventricular septal defect with pulmonary stenosis or atresia, dextrapostion of aorta, and hypertrophy of right ventricle. Valvular congenital anomalies of the heart include atresia and stenosis. Cor triatriatum (Q24.2) is when the heart has three atrial chambers with there being two left atriums. There can also be congenital malpositioning of the heart.

The great vessels of the heart can be transposed (Q20.3) including the superior and/or inferior vena cavae, pulmonary artery, pulmonary veins, and aorta. Other congenital anomalies can occur with the aorta and great veins, such as coarctation of aorta and anomaly of great veins (Q25.1). There are also congenital anomalies of the peripheral vascular system (Q27.8).

Section 22.5: RESPIRATORY

There are several congenital anomalies related to the respiratory system. This includes choanal atresia (Q30.0) when there is a growth of membrane or tissue over the nasal airways of the newborn. There are also congenital anomalies of missing or additional noses, or deformities to the nose. There can also be congenital anomalies of the larynx, trachea, and bronchus. Congenital cystic lung (Q33.0) can include bronchogenic cysts, benign mass of abnormal lung tissue, lobar emphysema, and pulmonary sequestration which is a mass of nonfunctioning pulmonary tissue.

Section 22.6: GASTROINTESTINAL/GENITOURINARY

CLEFT PALATE/LIP: A cleft is a fissure or opening of the palate or lip which usually occurs within the first couple months of gestation. Cleft palates/lips (Q35) are differentiated within the codes as to whether one or both conditions exist and if they are bilateral or unilateral and complete or incomplete. If the defect extends into the nose, then it is complete, but if it does not extend up into the nose, then it is incomplete.

OTHER GI/GU CONGENITAL ANOMALIES: Aglossia (Q38.3) is the absence of a tongue. Ankyloglossia (Q38.1) is known as tongue tied and is when the frenulum is unusually short which is the membrane connecting the underside of the tongue to the floor of the mouth. Hypertrophy of the tongue is known as macroglossia (Q38.2) and underdevelopment is known as microglossia.

Absence, stenosis, stricture, atresia, or fistulas can also occur of various anatomic sites of the GI/GU systems. A hernia can also be congenital (Q40.1). Meckel's diverticulum (Q43.0) is a small bulge in the small intestine present at birth. Congenital anomalies of the gallbladder, bile ducts, and liver include atresia, absence, duplication, and cysts.

Pyloric stenosis (Q40.0) occurs when there is narrowing of the opening to the stomach and hypertrophy of the pylorus (muscle surrounding the opening of the stomach). This results in severe vomiting in the first few months after birth. Other codes include congenital malformations, atresia, and absences of various parts of the digestive system.

Congenital anomalies of the GU system include conditions with the genital organs (Q50-Q56), such as absences, cysts, accessory anatomic parts, doubling of the uterus, undescended testicles, hypospadias, and indeterminate sex/hermaphroditism (Q56). Hypospadias is when the opening of the penis is located other than at the tip, such as on the underside. Hermaphroditism is having both female and male sex organs.

Polycystic kidney disease (Q61.3) is clusters of fluid-filled cysts in the kidneys which results in enlargement of the kidneys and replacement of kidney tissue which eventually results in uremia and kidney failure. It is further classified by being either autosomal dominant or recessive. To be dominant means that a child need only receive a defective gene from one parent because the gene is dominant and will cause the disease. With autosomal recessive, a child must receive the defective gene from both parents in order for the disease to exist. Another differentiation is if the disease is medullary. Medullary cystic kidney disease (Q61.5) is a hereditary disorder in which cysts in the center of each kidney cause the kidneys to gradually lose their ability to work. Medullary sponge kidney disease is a hereditary disorder in which there is formation of diffuse cysts in the center of the kidney caused by abnormalities in the renal collecting ducts.

Congenital obstruction of the kidneys and ureters are coded as to location (Q62). An ureterocele is a sac caused by the dilation of the ureters at the opening into the bladder. Exstrophy of the bladder occurs when the abdominal wall fails to close properly during development and the urinary bladder protrudes. Other anomalies include atresia and stenosis and fistulas and cysts.

Congenital abnormalities of the diaphragm (Q79.0) can include absence, hernia, or eventration. This code is not used for a congenital hiatal hernia; instead code Q40.1 should be used. Eventration is when all or part of the diaphragmatic muscle is replaced by fibroelastic tissue.

Section 22.7: MUSCULOSKELETAL

HIP: Congenital dislocation of the hip (Q65) are differentiated by being either unilateral or bilateral and defined as a dislocation or subluxation. Subluxation is an incomplete or partial dislocation.

LEGS: There are various curvature deformities of the leg that can occur congenitally. This includes genu extrorsum (bowleg) (Q68.3), genu introrsum (knock-knee) (Q74.1), genu recurvatum (hyperextensibility of the knee joint), genu valgum (knock-knee), and gen varum (bowleg).

FEET: Similar to acquired musculoskeletal deformities, deformities of the feet include talipes varus (Q66.0), talipes equinovarus (downward twisting of the foot), talipes valgus, and pes planus (Q66.5).

CHEST: Congenital chest deformities include pectus excavatum (Q67.6) and pectus carinatum. Excavatum is also known as funnel chest due to the malformation of the sternum and several ribs. Carinatum involves a pronunciation of the sternum. Other deformities can include more or less ribs than normal (supernumerary or absence Q76).

EXTREMITIES: Congenital anomalies of the extremities include polydactyly which is extra fingers or toes and syndactyly (Q70) when the fingers or toes grow together (webbed). Syndactyly can include fusion of bone. Other deformities include having fewer fingers or toes than a person should (reduction). Reduction can also include absence of other anatomic sites of the extremities including hands, feet, humerus, and femur. Reduction can be complete or incomplete depending upon if the entire anatomic site is missing or only partially missing. In addition, while one anatomic site may be missing, anatomic sites distal from that, such as fingers which are distal to the rest of the arm, may still exist. Abnormal growth of cartilage (chondrodystrophy Q77.3) can affect the limbs and affect the growth plates.

SPINE: Spina bifida (Q76.0) is a defective closure of the vertebral column and ranges in severity from occulta with few signs to completely open (rachischisis). In spina bifida occulta the outer part of some of the vertebrae are not completely closed but there is no protrusion of the spinal cord externally. Spina bifida is classified by whether hydrocephalus is involved or not. Hydrocephalus is the accumulation of cerebrospinal fluid within the ventricles of the brain. The affected area is designated by the fifth character. In spina bifida cystica, there is a protruding sac known as meningocele (involves meninges), myelocele (involves spinal cord), or myelomeningocele (involves both meninges and spinal cord). Paralysis can occur if the nerve roots are involved which is frequent. Spondylolisthesis is displacement of vertebrae.

BONE: Osteodystrophies (Q78) are bone anomalies including osteogenesis imperfecta which is when bones break easily. Osteopetrosis is when the bones are denser or harder and is known as stone bone. Osteopoikilosis is an asymptomatic osteosclerotic dysplasia of the bones. Polyostotic fibrous dysplasia of bone is the abnormal replacement of bone with scar-like tissue.

Section 22.8: INTEGUMENTARY

Congenital integumentary anomalies include edema (Q82), ichthyosis (wide variety of skin disorders characterized by dry, thickened, scaly or flaky skin), and dermatoglyphic anomalies which are abnormalities in the creases/prints of fingers, palms, toes, and soles. Birthmarks, strawberry nevus, and port-wine stains on the skin are coded as vascular hematomas (Q82.5).

Other pigmentary anomalies include urticaria pigmentosa, poikiloderma, skin tags and keratoderma. Urticaria pigmentosa is due to an excessive numbers of mast cells in the skin that produce hives. Poikiloderma is extra pigmentation of the skin. Keratoderma is thickening of the skin of the palms and soles, sometimes with painful fissuring.

Congenital anomalies of the hair (Q84) include alopecia (loss of hair), atrichosis and hypertrichosis is the absence or overgrowth of hair, respectively.

Congenital anomalies of nails (Q84.3) include anonychia (absence of nails), clubnail (increased curvature and thickening of nails), koilonychia (also known as spoon nails and the opposite of clubnails in that the nails are thinner and have decreased curvature), pachyonychia (excess keratin in nail beds and thickening of the nails with lesions), and leukonychia (white discoloration of nails).

Other integumentary congenital anomalies can include the absence or accessory breasts.

Section 22.9: CHROMOSOMAL

Chromosomal anomalies (Q90) include Down's syndrome which is also known as Mongolism or Trisomy 21 due to the nature of the genetic defect in which there are three 21st chromosomes, rather than the normal two. There are a wide variety of symptoms which is also true for Patau's syndrome (Trisomy 13) (Q91). Edward's Syndrome is also known as Trisomy E for there are three chromosomes for the 18th.

Other chromosomal anomalies include Cri-du-chat syndrome (Q93.4) and Klinefelter's Syndrome (Q98.4). Klinefelter's Syndrome occurs when a male has two X chromosomes and one Y instead of one Y and one X.

Section 22.10: OTHER CONGENITAL ANOMALIES

Other congenital anomalies include situs inversus (Q89.3) in which all of the major thoracic and abdominal organs are reversed horizontally, conjoined twins (Q89.4), and Prader-Willi syndrome in which there is a defect in the 15th chromosome which results in short stature with mental retardation and obesity. Marfan Syndrome is characterized by very tall stature with long limbs in addition to serious other anomalies of the heart and other organs. Fragile X syndrome (Q99.2) has a wide variety of characteristics also, including a long face and big ears with low muscle tone.

CONGENITAL QUIZ 16

1) What are the codes for a newborn who was born with a hemangioma of the neck?

2) What are the codes for a patient with lateral epicondylitis due to crushing injury?

3) What are the codes for a fetus at 35 weeks gestation who is diagnosed with a myelocele and spina bifida of C2-4 and hydrocephalus?

4) What are the codes for a newborn during this visit with congenital toxoplasmosis with hydrocephalus?

5) What are the codes for a fetus who has been diagnosed with Tetralogy of Fallot?

6) What are the codes for a missed abortion before 22 weeks for the mother?

7) What are the codes for an 8-year-old who is seen today for clubfoot that has developed over time?

8) What are the codes for a pregnant woma n whose baby has been diagnosed with Down's Syndrome?

9) What are the codes for a 3-day old baby who remains in the hospital after birth due to a diagnosis of Fallot's triad?

10) What are the codes for a 30-week pregnant woman with aplastic anemia?

11) What at the codes for a patient who has traumatic asphyxiation?

12) What are the codes for a 44-year-old man who has arthritis of his shoulder due to Lyme disease?

13) What are the codes for a 2-year-old child who has been diagnosed with congential hypothyroidism?

14) What are the codes for a baby born on this visit via C-section with fetal alcohol syndrome due to her mother's alcoholism and occasional cocaine?

13. What are the codes when a 1750 gm baby at 28 weeks gestation is delivered due to hypertonic labor?

CHAPTER 23
ICD-10 SYMPTOMS AND ILL-DEFINED CONDITIONS

You will learn the following objectives in this chapter:

A. Symptoms/ Signs
B. Circulatory/Respiratory
C. Digestive
D. Skin
E. Nervous/Musculoskeletal
F. Genitourinary
G. Emotional/Cognition
H. Speech
I. General Symptoms
J. Abnormal Findings

Chapter 18 is described as "Symptoms, Signs and Abnormal Clinical and Laboratory Findings, not elsewhere classified" and ranges from R00-R99. The symptoms and sign codes are specified by systems, such as R00-R09 is for circulatory and respiratory systems. Abnormal findings are based on content of examination, such as R70-R79 for blood work.

Section 23.1: SYMPTOMS/SIGNS

Symptoms are the descriptions provided by patients about their conditions, in other words they are subjective. In contrast, a sign is objective in that it is a condition that is present and observable.

SCENARIOS: There are three coding scenarios for symptoms and signs:

(1) Symptoms and signs are not coded if a definitive diagnosis is described.
(2) A sign and/or symptom may be coded in addition to a diagnosis that includes them if the sign and/or symptom requires treatment and attention, such as dehydration.
(3) If there is no definitive diagnosis described that would include the signs and/or symptoms, then the signs and/or symptoms would be coded.
(4) If the diagnosis is described as provisional (that is probable, possible, rule out, etc.), then the diagnosis is not coded but the sign and/or symptom would be instead.

Section 23.2: CIRCULATORY/RESPIRATORY

Symptoms and signs associated with circulatory include tachycardia (R00.0) and bradycardia (R00.1). Additional symptoms include palpitations, murmurs, and abnormal blood-pressure readings. Respiratory symptoms include hemorrhages (R04), cough (R05), dyspnea (R06.0) which is difficulty breathing including shortness of breath, stridor, wheezing, hiccoughs and sneezing. Apnea, tachypnea, and snoring are coded as R06.8 codes. Pain in the throat and chest are coded as R07. Asphyxia, hypoxemia, pleurisy, respiratory arrest, and postnasal drip are coded as R09 codes.

Section 23.3: DIGESTIVE

Symptoms and signs associated with the digestive system include abdominal and pelvic pain (R10) which is differentiated by which quadrant the pain is located in. It is important to be sure to be precise in the selection of codes because the codes are specific, e.g. pain in the stomach and abdomen are coded differently. Abdominal tenderness (R10.8) is differentiated by the presence or absence of rebounding. Colic is coded as R10.83. Nausea and vomiting (R11) is differentiated as to type, such as projective or bilious. Heartburn is coded as R12.

Other symptoms of the digestive system include aphagia and dysphagia. Be careful because this is phagia (associated with eating), not phasia (associated with speaking). Flatulence is coded as R14 and includes gas pain, eructation and distension.

Hepatomegaly and splenomegaly are coded as R16 if not classified elsewhere. Ascites is coded as R18. Swelling, mass or lump in the abdominal area is coded as R19.0 and is differentiated by quadrant of the body. Abnormal bowel sounds are coded as R19.1 and include absent or hyperactive. Abdominal rigidity (R19.3) is differentiated by quadrant location.

Section 23.4: SKIN

Symptoms associated with the skin include skin sensation (R20) such as anesthesia (no feeling), hypoesthesia (reduced feeling), paresthesia (tingling feeling), and hyperesthesia (increased feeling). Swelling, mass or lump of the skin is coded as R22 and differentiated by specific location.

Skin changes (R23) can include cyanosis, pallor, flushing or ecchymoses.

Section 23.5: NERVOUS & MUSCULOSKELETAL

Nervous symptoms include abnormal involuntary movements (R25) such as tremors, cramps, spasms, or fasciculations. Mobility symptoms (R26) include ataxic or paralytic gait and unsteadiness. Ataxia is coded as R27.0.

Other symptoms include tetany, clicking hip, repeated falls, facial weakness, loss of height and ocular torticollis.

Section 23.6: GENITOURINARY

Symptoms associated with the genitourinary system (R30-R39) include dysuria and painful micturition. Hematuria (R31) is differentiated as gross, benign or other. Retention of urine (R33) can be due to drugs or other causes such as enlarged prostate. Anuria and oliguria are coded as R34 and polyuria as R35.

Section 23.7: EMOTIONAL AND COGNITION

Symptoms coded in this section (R40-R46) include somnolence, stupor, and coma.

Comas are differentiated by responses and the Glasgow scale. There is a box listing the possible seventh character values similar to the boxes in the ICD-9 book. The coding with the Glasgow coma scale is accomplished by the selection of one code from each of R40.21 (Coma scale, eyes open), R40.22 (coma scale, best verbal response), and R40.23 (coma scale, best motor response). These codes (R40.21 – R40.23) are only used if the individual scores are given for the responses. If only a total score is given for the Glasgow coma scale, then codes R40.24 should be used. Responses can include various levels associated with the following: eyes open, verbal or motor response. A seventh character needs to be added to specify when the coma scale was completed.

Other symptoms include disorientation, amnesia, neglect, age-related, borderline intellectual functioning, and dizziness. Disturbances of smell and taste are coded as R43 and include anosmia, parosmia and parageusia. Hallucinations are coded as R44 and can be auditory, visual or other. Codes for emotional states (R45) include nervousness, unhappiness, restlessness, demoralization, apathy, hostility, irritability, low self-esteem, worries, excessive crying of child, and homicidal or suicidal ideation.

Section 23.8: SPEECH

Symptoms associated with speech and voice (R47-R49) include dysphasia, aphasia, slurred speech, dysarthria, dyslexia, apraxia, dysphonia, aphonia, and hypernasality.

Section 23.9: GENERAL SYMPTOMS

General symptoms (R50-R69) include fever of unknown origin or post-procedural. Headache is coded as R51. Malaise and fatigue are coded as R53 and include functional quadriplegia. Age-related debility is coded as R54 and includes frailty, old age, senile, and senescence. Syncope includes collapse, blackout, or fainting. Convulsions are coded as (R56) and can be febrile or post-traumatic. Shock not coded elsewhere is coded as R57 and include cardiogenic and hypovolemic.

Other general symptoms include enlarged lymph nodes (R59), edema (R60), delayed milestones for development as child (R62.0), failure to thrive as a child (R62.51), short stature ((R62.52), and food/fluid problems such as anorexia, polydipsia, polyphagia, abnormal weight loss or gain and cachexia which is wasting syndrome.

Sepsis codes are coded as R65 codes including systemic inflammatory response syndrome (SIRS) and severe sepsis. Severe sepsis codes list the various associated conditions that would define the sepsis as severe such as shock or organ failure which should also be coded.

Other generalized codes include excessive crying by a baby (R68.11), dry mouth (R68.2) and clubbing of fingers (R68.3).

Section 23.10: ABNORMAL FINDINGS

Nonspecific Abnormal Findings (R70-R79) are codes when labs and tests findings are not normal but not enough information is known to determine a diagnosis.

Abnormal findings codes should not be listed unless the physician states they are abnormal and that no other diagnosis is available for those findings. Other qualified practitioners can also provide valid diagnosis and /or conditions, such as pathologist and laboratory technicians who are qualified. Abnormal findings should be not listed if they are not pertinent to the care of the patient at this visit.

Abnormal findings can include abnormalities in red blood cells (R71), glucose (R73.0), alcohol blood levels (R78.0), inconclusive tests for HIV (R75), increased antibodies (R76), presence of drugs (R78), and blood chemistries (R79).

Abnormal findings on urine tests are coded as R80-R82 and can include proteinuria, biluria (urine which contains bile pigments), hemoglobinuria, and glycosuria.

Other abnormal labs (R83-R89) can include specimens such as from cerebrospinal fluid, respiratory organs, digestive organs, PAP smear, genitourinary, and hemodialysis.

Abnormal findings from diagnostic tests such as x-rays (R90-R94) are differentiated by the anatomic site as well as function tests.

Abnormal tumor markers are coded as R97 and demonstrate presence of antigen such as for cancer and prostate.

SYMPTOMS QUIZ 17

1) What are the codes for a 4-year-old patient with high fever, sore throat, and runny nose who is found to have acute right otitis media with rhinitis?

2) What are the codes for a patient with pathological fracture of the distal radius and COPD with Type I diabetes?

3) What are the codes for a patient who is 82-years-old and broke her right hip and has been severely depressed since?

4) What are the codes for a patient with second and third degree burns covering 25% of her body with 10% being third degree with infection?

5) What are the codes for a pregnant patient who ws seen for vaginal bleeding at 20 weeks gestation and she had three prior spontaneous abortions at this same time in the pregnancy?

6) What are the codes for a patient who underwent chemotherapy today for small cell carcinoma lung cancer and is now experiencing vomiting without nausea?

14. What are the codes for a patient who has old bucket tear of the lateral meniscus?

7) What are the codes for a patient with an infected wound of the right humerus which was greenstick fractured with a dislocation and laceration of the axillary nerves?

8) What are the codes for a patient with stage 5 renal disease and hypertension as well as arteriolar nephritis and chronic hypertensive uremia?

9) What are the codes for a 45-year-old man with shortness of breath?

10) What are the codes for a patient with scar tissue of his chest from a third degree burn six months ago?

11) What are the codes for a patient with complaints of dyspnea and tachycardia which the physician believes might be ARDS?

12) What are the codes for a patient with acute and chronic bronchitis with COPD and ASHD?

13) What are the codes for a 72-year-old man who is seen for elevated liver function studies but hepatitis profile and sugar levels were normal? He is also diabetic Type 2 and has cholelithiasis.

14) What are the codes for a 57-year-old man who was admitted to the hospital for possible MI with complaints of chest pain with numbness of the left arm? EKG and stress tests were performed but were negative.

CHAPTER 24
ICD-10 INJURIES, POISONING & CERTAIN OTHER CONSEQUENCES

You will learn the following objectives in this chapter:

A. Injuries
B. Fractures
    1. Closed Fractures
    2. Open Fractures
    3. Malunion/Nonunion
    4. Extensions
    5. Pathological Fractures
    6. Dislocations
C. Sprains/Strains
D. Superficial
E. Open wounds
F. Hemorrhage/Hematoma
G. Vessels/Nerves
H. Head/Skull
I. Neck
J. Thorax
K. Abdomen/Pelvis/Genitals
L. Shoulder/Upper Arms
M. Wrist/Hands/Fingers
N. Hip/Thigh
O. Knee/Lower Leg
P. Ankle/Foot/Toes
Q. Injury/Poisoning/Other
R. Foreign Body
S. Burns
    1. Degrees
    2. Lund Browder Chart
    3. Percentage
T. Frostbite
U. Poisonings/Adverse Effects
    1. Underdosing
    2. Table of Drugs and Chemicals
    3. Coding for Adverse Effects
    4. Coding for Poisonings
    5. Coding for Underdosings
V. Toxic Effects
W. Other Conditions
X. Early Complications of Trauma
Y. Complications of Medical Care

Chapter 19 is described as "Injury, Poisoning, and Certain Other Consequences of External Causes" and ranges from S00-T88. S codes are specific to body regions and T codes are specific to unspecified body regions. There is a significantly increased number of codes in this section. Injuries are now organized according to anatomic site, with injuries listed secondary.

Section 24.1: INJURIES

The first block of codes are first differentiated by anatomic site and then by injury. Injury is bodily damage or injury caused by an external force (trauma). Types of injuries include superficial and open wounds, burns, fractures, dislocation, crushing, bites, rupture, foreign bodies, bruises, sprain/strains, and amputations. Injuries to organs, muscles, tendons, vessels, and nerves are also listed within each anatomic site.

Codes are now highly specific to site such as which finger or toe and laterality (left or right).

If there are multiple injuries, the most severe injury should be listed first.

An extra seventh character is added for injuries and external causes to identify the encounter as initial, subsequent, or sequelae. The extensions are:

- A Initial encounter
- D Subsequent encounter
- S Sequelae

Late effects are coded using the extension S for sequelae.

Section 24.2: FRACTURES

Fractures are a break in the continuity of the bone which can be caused by trauma or a disease process.

- Open fracture is one in which the skin was broken and there is exposure to the outside which creates a possibility of infection or other complications by the entry of foreign materials into the body.
- Closed fracture is when there is no breakage of skin.

- Complete fractures are fractures in which bone fragments separate completely.
- Incomplete fractures are fractures in which the bone fragments are still partially joined.
- Compacted fractures are fractures caused when bone fragments are driven into each other.
- Stress fractures are caused by unusual or repeated stress on a bone.
- Compression fractures are fractures of the vertebrae where the front portion of a vertebra in the spine collapses.
- Le Fort fractures are bilateral horizontal fracture of the maxilla. Le Fort fractures are classified as I, II, or III.

- Monteggia's fracture is a fracture of the proximal half of the shaft of the ulna, with dislocation of the head of the radius.

CLOSED FRACTURES

- Simple fractures are fractures that only occur along one line, splitting the bone into two pieces.
- Depressed fractures are fractures of the skull in which a fragment is depressed.
- Elevated fractures are when fractured portion is elevated above the level of the intact skull.
- Fissured fractures are cracks extending from a surface into, but not through, a long bone.
- Greenstick fracture are fractures in which one side of a bone is broken, the other being bent.
- Impacted fractures are fractures in which one fragment is firmly driven into the other.
- Slipped capital epiphysis fractures are separations of the ball of the hip joint from the femur at the upper growing end of the bone.
- Comminuted fractures are fractures in which there are multiple pieces.
- Linear fractures are fractures that are parallel to the bone's long axis.
- Transverse fractures are fractures that are at a right angle to the bone's long axis.
- Oblique fractures are fractures that are diagonal to a bone's long axis.
- Spiral fractures are fractures where at least one part of the bone has been twisted.

OPEN FRACTURES: The following terms indicate that the skin has been broken:
- Compound fractures are open fractures in which the skin is broken.
- Infected fractures are open fractures in which foreign bodies which   gained access through the open wound have caused an infection.
- Missile, puncture, foreign body indicates fractures in which the skin has been broken by an external object.

The seventh character denotes if the fracture is open or closed for an initial encounter or if a subsequent encounter is for routine healing, delayed healing, nonunion, malunion, or sequelae. A malunion means the fracture did not heal together properly. A nonunion means the fracture did not heal together at all.

The fracture extensions are:

- A Initial encounter for closed fracture
- B Initial encounter for open fracture
- D Subsequent encounter for fracture with routine healing
- G Subsequent encounter for fracture with delayed healing
- K Subsequent encounter for fracture with nonunion
- S Sequelae

Subsequent is used for encounters after the patient has received active treatment of an injury whereas sequelae is used for complications or conditions that result from an injury such as scar tissue from a burn.

Like the ICD-9 codes, if there is no description of the fracture being open or closed, it is coded as closed. If the fracture is not described as displaced or nondisplaced, then it should be coded as displaced. In a displaced fracture, the two ends of the bone are separated from each other.

Do not use Z codes for aftercare of injuries as the aftercare for injuries is care provided during the healing process and the regular S or T code should be used for the injury itself.

PATHOLOGICAL FRACTURE: If a fracture is caused by a disease process, then the fracture is described as pathological and this term should be included in the selection of the proper codes which are not coded from these codes but rather from M84 codes.

DISLOCATIONS: While fractures and dislocations can be coded separately, when they occur together as an injury, i.e. fracture/dislocation, the fracture codes are now differentiated based on if there is a dislocation or not. Dislocations (also known as displacements or subluxation) should be coded when present if they are the only injury. A subluxation is a partial dislocation.

Dislocations are classified by anatomic sites and if they are open or closed. Dislocations can be either open or closed based also on the premise that there is a break in the skin which would be open. However, closed dislocations may be described as complete, NOS, simple, partial or uncomplicated. Open dislocations are described as compound, infected, or with foreign body. Dislocation of knees include tears of cartilage or meniscus which includes bucket handle tears. Dislocations of knees are also classified by area, i.e., anterior, posterior, medial or lateral.

Although similar to dislocations, derangements are a chronic condition in which the anatomic site has become disarranged and should be coded with musculoskeletal codes (M codes) because they are not traumatic injuries.

Section 24.3: SPRAINS/STRAINS

A sprain is an injury of the ligaments when they are stretched beyond their normal capacity and possibly torn. Whiplash is a sprain of the cervical spine. Strains are a similar injury to sprains, but they occur to muscles and tendons. Sprains and strains codes also include avulsions, hemarthrosis, laceration, rupture and tears of joint capsules, ligaments, muscles, and tendons. If these occur in an open wound, then this is coded as an open wound. Sprains and strains are classified by anatomic site and part, i.e., ligament, tendon, etc. Whiplash is coded as S13.4.

Section 24.4: SUPERFICIAL

Superficial injuries include abrasions, friction burns, blisters, insect bites, superficial foreign body, and others. An abrasion is superficial damage to the skin not extending beyond the epidermis and is not as severe as a laceration. An avulsion is a traumatic abrasion that removes all layers of skin. Blister is a pocket of fluid in the epidermis and dermis oftentimes caused by friction, burning, infection, freezing, and chemical exposure.

Superficial injuries do not include burns, contusions, foreign bodies, venomous insect bites, and open wound which are coded with T codes and will be discussed later. Superficial injuries are further classified by anatomic site and infected or not infected. Contusions with intact skin include bruising or hematoma without fracture or open wound.

Crushing injury are classified by anatomic site. Any additional injuries should also be coded, such as fracture, internal or intracranial injuries.

Section 24.5: OPEN WOUNDS

Open wounds are also known as lacerations. A wound is an injury to the soft tissue in conjunction with an interruption of the skin. Wounds may be described as incising, puncturing and penetrating. Penetrating indicates the passage of an object into or through the body. If there is an accumulation of blood in a body cavity due the wound, this is known as a hemothorax, hemopericardium, hemoperitoneum, or hemoarthrosis based on which cavity is involved. Open wounds include animal bites, avulsions, cut, laceration, punctures, amputations, and trauma.

Wounds are not coded if they are associated with a more serious injury, such as a fracture or internal injury.

A complicated wound is indicated as having delayed healing, delayed treatment, foreign body, or infection present. Infection of wounds is now coded as an additional code rather than included as part of the description of the wound as complicated.

Section 24.6: HEMORRHAGE/HEMATOMA

Hemorrhage is bleeding. Hematoma is a collection of blood outside the blood vessels, otherwise known as internal bleeding. A subdural hematoma occurs between the dura and the leptomeninges of the brain. Subarachnoid hematoma or hemorrhage occurs directly beneath the arachnoid.

Contusions are soft tissue injuries in which the skin is not broken but there is bleeding within which results in a hematoma. Hemorrhages and hematomas are specified according to the part of the brain involved, type of injury, and level of consciousness.

Section 24.7: VESSELS/NERVES

Traumatic injury to vessels and nerves are coded within each anatomic site. This includes avulsions, hematomas, laceration, rupture, fistula, and aneurysm. These codes are classified by the vessel and nerve involved. Remember that with the spinal cord, injuries are classified by the interspace between two vertebrae, i.e., C1-C3 is two interspaces, C1-C2 and C2-C3.

Section 24.8: HEAD/SKULL

Injuries to the head are coded as S00-S09. There should be an additional code listed if there is an infection also. This section also includes traumatic injuries to the eye, ear, nose, and lips. Any injuries to nerves or vessels should be coded in addition. Superficial foreign body injuries and bites by nonvenomous insects are coded in these sections. These types of injuries are included in each anatomic site within the injury codes

Superficial injuries of the head and all areas including eyes and ears are coded as S00. Open wounds of the head are coded as S01 which includes bites, puncture wounds, and lacerations.

A laceration (wound) is when there is a traumatic disruption of skin. A contusion is a closed wound and is more serious than a concussion as it is damage to the brain in the form of a bruise with bleeding.

Fractures of the skull (S02) are differentiated by anatomic site of the skull, and type of encounter. Additional codes (S06) should be coded if patient was unconscious. A blowout fracture is a fracture of the walls or floor of the orbit (eye socket) with fragments possibly pushed into the paranasal sinuses.

The section of codes (S06) for intracranial injuries do not include those with skull fractures which were coded with S02 codes. All intracranial injuries are classified by loss of consciousness within each type of traumatic injury. They are differentiated by the length of time the person experiences loss of consciousness, i.e., less than 30 minutes (S06.0X1) or 31 to 59 minutes (S06.0X2) and so forth for longer periods of time using S06 codes. Seventh digits indicate if it is initial encounter (A), subsequent encounter (D) or sequela (S).

A concussion is coded as S06.0. Edema of the brain caused by trauma is coded as S06.1. Other types of brain injury include diffuse, focal, contusions, lacerations, and hemorrhage and are highly differentiated by specific anatomic site.

Crushing injuries of the head are coded as S07 and include face and skull. Amputations are coded as S08. Injuries to blood vessels, tendons, and muscles of the head are coded as S09 and specific to anatomic site and laterality.

Section 24.9: NECK

Codes for the neck and trunk (S10 – S19) include the vertebrae. Superficial injuries and open wounds are coded as S10-S11. Spinal cord injuries should be coded additionally as well as infection.

As with most spinal cord codes (S12), the location of the fracture on the spinal column should be coded for cervical in this section. These codes are also further differentiated by whether the fracture is open or closed and displaced or nondisplaced. Remember to code as closed or displaced if type not known. If there is spinal cord injury, then the codes are differentiated by what part of the cord is involved, that is the anterior or central cord. The codes also distinguish if there is a lesion or not (lesion is damage or injury).

Dislocation and sprain of joints and ligaments are coded as S13. This includes avulsions, lacerations, sprains, hemoarthrosis, rupture, tear, and subluxation. These codes are differentiated by the two vertebrae involved and comprising the intervertebral space, such as C1-C2 which counts as one diagnosis.

Injuries of nerves and spinal cord in the neck area are coded as S14. This includes concussion, edema, lesions, cord syndrome, and injuries. Injuries of blood vessels are coded as S15 as differentiated by specific artery involved. Injury of muscles, fascia and tendons are coded as S16 which include strains and lacerations.

Crushing injuries of the neck area are coded as S17.

Section 24.10: THORAX

Pneumothorax is also known as a collapsed lung when air or gas is able to enter the pleural cavity due to trauma or disease. Hemothorax is when blood accumulates in the pleural cavity. Injuries to the thorax area (S20-S29) include superficial, contusions, blisters, abrasions, superficial bites, nonvenomous insect bites, and external constrictions. With open wounds (S21) any associated injury should be coded such as hemopneumothorax or fractures. Some of these codes are differentiated as to whether there was penetration into the thoracic cavity.

Fractures of the ribs, sternum, and thoracic spine are coded as S22. Again, if the type is not known, then fractures should be coded as closed and/or displaced. As with the cervical vertebrae, the specific vertebrae should be listed. Flail chest (S22.5) occurs when there are multiple fractures of the ribs and sternum which causes the chest to be unstable.

Dislocation and subluxation of joints and ligaments of the thorax, as well as injuries to nerves and spinal cord are coded as S23 and differentiated by intervertebral space, i.e. T1-T2. Injuries to blood vessels are coded as S25 and differentiated by vessel involved.

Injuries to the heart are coded as S26 and any hemothorax and/or pneumothorax should be coded additionally.

Injuries to other intrathoracic organs are coded as S27 including lungs, bronchus, thoracic part of the trachea and esophagus, pleura, and diaphragm.

Crushing chest injuries are coded as S28.0. Traumatic amputation of part of the thorax is coded as S28.2 and can include the breast.

Injuries to muscles and tendons are coded as S29.

Section 24.11: ABDOMEN/PELVIS/GENITALS

Injuries to the abdomen, lower back, lumbar spine, pelvis and external genitals are coded as S30-S39.   These include blisters, contusions, external constriction, and superficial foreign body and bites by nonvenomous insects. Open wounds are coded as S31.

Injuries to the liver (S3) are classified based on the extent of the wound (minor, moderate or major) and if there is a hematoma and/or contusion. A laceration is considered minor if it extends less than 1 cm deep. A laceration is considered moderate if it extends to less than 3 cm deep but more than 1 cm. A laceration is considered major if it extends to more than 3 cm deep which significantly disrupts the parenchyma (functional parts of an organ).

Fracture of the lumbar spine and pelvis are coded as S32. They are differentiated by zones and types. Zone I is the most distal from the spinal cord and Zone III is the most proximal, central portion of the spinal cord. Types vary according to whether they are flexion or extension and with posterior or anterior displacement.

Dislocation and sprain of joints and ligaments of lumbar spine and pelvis are coded as S33 and include subluxation. Injury of lumbar and sacral spinal cord and nerves in the abdominal/pelvic area are coded as S34. All of these codes are differentiated by intervertebral segment involved which is denoted by the vertebrae involved such as L1-L2. Injuries of blood vessels in the abdominal/pelvic area are coded as S35.

Injury to internal organs in the abdominal area are coded as S36 and include spleen, gallbladder, bile ducts, pancreas, stomach, colon, rectum, and peritoneum. Codes for injury to the urinary and pelvic organs are coded with S37 codes and include the kidneys, ureter, ovary, bladder, urethra, fallopian tubes, uterus, and prostate.

Crushing injuries to abdominal/pelvic areas are coded as S38. Amputations are coded as S38.2. Injuries to muscle, fascia, and tendons are coded as S39.0.

Section 24.12: SHOULDER/UPPER ARM

Injuries of the shoulder and upper arm are coded as S40-S49. These include contusions, superficial foreign body, nonvenomous insect bites, wounds, laceration, dislocation, subluxation, sprain, and fractures. Injuries to the nerves are coded as S44 for the shoulder and S54 for the upper arm. Injury to blood vessels is coded as S45 for shoulder and S55 for the forearm. Injuries of muscles, fascia, and tendons are coded as S46 for the shoulder and S56. Crushing injuries are coded as S47 for the shoulder and S57 for the upper forearm. Amputations are coded as S48 for the shoulder and S58 for the upper forearm. Notice there are significantly more codes in these sections as they are very specific to exact anatomic sites and laterality.

Fractures of the forearm are coded as S52 and open fractures are differentiated by the Gustilo open fracture classification which is based on wound size, soft tissue contamination and damage, as well as if the fracture is comminuted or not.

Section 24.13: WRIST/HAND/FINGERS

Injuries to the wrist, hand and fingers are coded as S60-S69. As in the previous sections it includes codes for contusions, blisters, abrasion, nonvenomous insect bite, superficial foreign bodies, external constriction, open wound, amputation, fracture, dislocation, subluxation, traumatic rupture, crushing, and damage to nerves, vessels, tendons, muscles, fascia and tendons. The fracture codes also include the use of the Gustilo open fracture classification system.

Section 24.14: HIP/THIGH

Injuries to the hip and thigh are coded as S70-S79. As in the previous sections it includes codes for contusions, blisters, abrasion, nonvenomous insect bite, superficial foreign bodies, external constriction, open wound, amputation, fracture, dislocation, subluxation, traumatic rupture, crushing, and damage to nerves, vessels, tendons, muscles, fascia and tendons. The fracture codes also include the use of the Gustilo open fracture classification system.

Section 24.15: KNEE/LOWER LEG

Injuries to the knee and lower leg are coded as S80-S89. As in the previous sections it includes codes for contusions, blisters, abrasion, nonvenomous insect bite, superficial foreign bodies, external constriction, open wound, amputation, fracture, dislocation, subluxation, traumatic rupture, crushing, and damage to nerves, vessels, tendons, muscles, fascia and tendons. The fracture codes also include the use of the Gustilo open fracture classification system.

Section 24.16: ANKLE/FOOT/TOES

Injuries to the ankle, foot and toes are coded as S90-S99. As the previous sections it includes codes for contusions, blisters, abrasion, nonvenomous insect bite, superficial foreign bodies, external constriction, open wound, amputation, fracture, dislocation, subluxation, traumatic rupture, crushing, and damage to nerves, vessels, tendons, muscles, fascia and tendons. The fracture codes also include the use of the Gustilo open fracture classification system.

Section 24:17: INJURY, POISONING & OTHER

Injury to unspecified body regions are coded as T14 and include abrasions, contusions, fracture, and crushing. If there are multiple unspecified sites they are coded together as T07.

Section 24.18: FOREIGN BODY

Foreign bodies entering the body through a natural orifice are coded as T15-T19. T15 codes are for the eye, T16 for the ear, T17 for the respiratory tract, T18 for the alimentary tract (esophagus, stomach, intestine, colon, anus and rectum), and T19 for the genitourinary tract (urethra, bladder, vulva, vagina, uterus, and penis).

Section 24.19: BURNS

Burns are injury to the layers of the skin but can extend into other parts of the body, including muscles, bones, and blood vessels. Burns can occur due to many reasons, including chemical agents, trauma, radiation, and electrical currents.

DEGREES: Burns are classified by the extent of damage to the skin and underlying tissues.
- FIRST DEGREE: A first degree burn only involves the epidermis with no blisters.
- SECOND DEGREE: A second degree burn includes the epidermal and dermal layers (known as partial-thickness) of the skin and can include blistering and hyperesthesia.
- THIRD DEGREE: A third degree burn includes all layers of the skin with necrosis of the epidermis and dermis layers and damage to the subcutaneous layer.
- NECROSIS: Necrosis is the death of tissue which results from a serious burn.

If there are multiple degrees of burn at the one site, then the highest degree burn should be coded. A non-healing burn is coded as an acute burn. Necrosis is also considered a non-healing burn. If an infection is present, be sure to code it also. If the organism causing the infection is known, code that also.

LUND-BROWDER CHART: The Lund-Browder Chart is also known as the Rule of Nines which is the division of the parts of body into multiples of nine so that the percentage of the total body surface area burned can be determined. Percentages for an adult are: 9% for the head/neck (front and back), each arm 9%, each leg 18%, anterior trunk 18%, posterior trunk 18%, and genitalia 1%. With a child these percentages change because a child's head is bigger in comparison to their body with 17% for the head/neck (front and back), each arm 9%, each leg 13%, anterior trunk 18%, posterior trunk 18%, and genitalia 1%. For a child less than 10 kg, the total body surface area burned percentages are 20% for the head/neck (front and back), each arm 8%, each leg 16%, anterior trunk 16%, posterior trunk 16%, and genitalia 1%.

Injuries due to burns and corrosion are coded as T20-T32. These can occur due to electricity, flame, friction, hot air and gases, lightning, radiation and chemicals. Seventh characters are based on if the encounter is initial, subsequent, or if it is a sequela.

The external source of the burn, place and intent should also be coded using X00-X19, X75-X77, X96-X98, and Y92.

If the extent of the body surface burned is known, then codes T31 or T32 should also be listed.

Burns of unspecified degree are coded to specific anatomic sites. T20.0 are codes for burns of the head, face and neck. First degree burns of the head, face, and neck are coded as T20.1, second degree as T20.2, third degree as T20.3 and corrosion as T20.4. For the trunk, unspecified degree is coded as T21.0, first degree as T21.1, second as T21.1, third degree as T21.3, and corrosion as T21.4. Unspecified degrees of shoulder and arms (not including hands and wrist) are coded as T22.0, first degree as T22.1, second degree as T22.2, third degree as T22.3, and corrosion as T22.4. Unspecified degrees of wrist and hand are coded as T23.0, first degree as T23.1, second degree as T23.2, third degree as T23.3, and corrosion as T23.4. Unspecified degree burns of the leg except ankle and foot are coded as T24.0, first degree as T24.1, second degree as T24.2, third degree as T24.3, and corrosion as T24.4.

Burns of the eye and adnexa are coded as T26 and are differentiated by specific anatomic part of the eye and laterality and not degree. Burns of the respiratory tract are coded as T27 by specific anatomic site and laterality also and not degree.

PERCENTAGE: Extent of body surface burned is coded as T31 and is based on percentage of body burned. The fourth character indicates the percentage of total body surface burned including all degrees. The fifth character indicates the percentage of body surface that was third degree burns.

Section 24.20: FROSTBITE

Frostbite is coded as T33-T34. It is differentiated by anatomic site, laterality, and if it is superficial or involving necrosis of tissue.

Section 24.21: POISONINGS/ADVERSE EFFECTS

Poisonings, adverse effect and underdosing are now included together in one code so no additional codes are needed. Poisonings are differentiated as accidental, intentional self-harm, assault, undetermined, or underdosing. They are coded as T36-T50 and are specific to drug, medicaments or biological substances involved. If the intent in the taking of the substance is not known, then it should be coded as accidental.

POISONING: Poisoning and underdosing codes are differentiated by the same methods as in the ICD-9, i.e. if the substance was taken as a poisoning or if it was taken properly but the patient suffered an adverse effect.

A poisoning occurs when a toxic substance, such as drugs or chemicals, is swallowed, inhaled, or comes in contact with the skin, eyes, or mucous membranes, resulting in harmful effects but the substance was not taken according to a physician's recommendations. Poisonings can occur due to numerous reasons:
- First, the patient may have chosen to overdose, possibly in an attempt to commit suicide.
- Second, the patient may have taken another person's prescriptions.
- Third, a wrong dosage may have been given erroneously by medical care personnel.
- Fourth, someone may have provided the substance to a person for the reasons of murder.
- Fifth, the patient may have mixed up medications, whether their own or someone else's.
- Sixth, the patient may have taken a prescription drug in combination with alcohol as alcohol with any prescription is not in accordance with medical advice.

- Seventh, the patient may have taken a prescription with an over-the-counter which they did not tell the physician they were taking, and the combination has detrimental effects.
- Eighth, the patient may have taken the wrong amount.
- Ninth, wrong dosage given by a non-medical person.

ADVERSE EFFECT: An adverse effect is when a patient takes a substance, such as drugs, in accordance with doctor's orders, but the patient still experiences a harmful reaction. Adverse effects can occur due to numerous reasons.

- First, this include toxicity wherein the patient took the substance or drug as recommended but for various reasons it was too strong for the person and caused an adverse effect. This may be due to an inappropriate level prescribed for the patient or the occurrence of a cumulative effect in which previous drugs or substances compounded the strength of the substance.
- Second, the patient may have suffered a hypersensitivity, allergic reaction, to the substance.
- Third, a synergistic effect may have occurred in which one substance heightens the effect of another substance.
- Fourth, one substance may interact inappropriately with another substance.
- Fifth, various side effects are always associated with substances.

UNDERDOSING: Underdosing occurs when a person takes less of a medication than prescribed or instructed by manufacturer or healthcare provider. Additional codes should be provided for all manifestations and for intent such as failure in dosage during medical care (Y63.61, Y63.8-Y63.9) and patient's underdosing of medication regime (Z91.12, Z91.13).

TABLE OF DRUGS AND CHEMICALS: The Table of Drugs and Chemicals follows the Alphabetical Index and Neoplasm Table. It is known as Alphabetical Index to Poisoning and External Causes of Adverse Effects of Drugs and Chemical Substances. It is broken into columns for poisonings, underdosing, and adverse effects with T codes. It contains a listing of drugs and chemicals with categories based on their means of introduction into the body. The headings are: Poisoning Accidental, Poisoning Intentional, Poisoning Assault, Poisoning Undetermined, Adverse effect and Underdosing.

This table lists various substances that can adversely affect someone, including legal and illegal drugs, toxins, cleaning supplies, poisons, chemicals, prescriptions, environmental toxins, etc.

The substances are listed by generic and brand names, but not all brand names are listed. In such a case when the brand name cannot be found, generic name must be used. Generic names are the scientific names for the drugs and the brand names are the names provided by manufacturers to distinguish their product from other manufacturers' products. The first letter of a brand name drug is capitalized, but not for a generic name.

There are several ways to find the generic name for a brand name drug that is not listed.

- First, if you know the generic name is ibuprofen for the brand name Advil, then you can look for ibuprofen in the Table of Drugs and Chemicals.

- Second, if you do not know the generic name, you can search for it in Appendix C which is the Classification of Drugs by AHFS List.
- Third, and perhaps an easier way, is to find the brand name in a drug book, such as the PDR, or search for it on the internet and the generic will be listed there.

CODING FOR ADVERSE EFFECTS: Adverse effect scenarios are only used when the patient has taken the substance in accordance with medical advice and experienced side effects. . When a patient has taken a substance properly and in accordance with medical advice, yet they experienced an adverse effect, then the adverse effect is listed first (such as gastritis) which is a regular code. Then the T code for the drug would be listed. Code as many substances involved.

CODING FOR POISONINGS: For coding of poisonings, the poisoning code should be listed first. Remember, you will provide codes for each substance involved. There are several coding scenarios for poisonings:
- First, a condition may be described as well as the substance causing the poisoning. In this case, the condition is listed first and then the poisoning code.
- Second, a condition may be present in addition to a prescription drug, but the person may have ingested over-the-counter drugs without informing the physician; therefore, this is against medical advice and so a poisoning code is assigned to each substance. Be sure to code the over-the-counter drug as well.
- Third, a condition may be present in addition to a prescription drug as well as alcohol which is always against medical advice and so this should be coded as a poisoning for both the prescription and the alcohol.

Poisoning codes include T36-T50. The various codes are differentiated by type of drugs, medicaments and biological substance. T36 is to be used for poisonings involving antibiotics. Poisonings by hormones is coded as T38. Poisonings by narcotics is coded as T40. Poisonings by anesthetics is coded as T41. Poisonings by agents affecting the gastrointestinal system are coded as T47.

CODING FOR UNDERDOSING: Under-dosing is described as taking less of a medication than is prescribed by physician either purposely or by mistake. Intent of the underdosing should be also be coded such as failure in dosage during medical care (Y63.61) or patient's underdosing (Z91.12).

Section 24.22: TOXIC EFFECTS

Codes for toxic effects due to a substance include T51 to T65. T51 is for toxic effect of alcohol. Toxic effects of corrosive substances is coded as T54. Toxic effects of soap and detergents is coded as T55. Toxic effects of metals is coded as T56. Toxic effects of gases and fumes is coded as T59. Toxic effects from contact with venomous animals and plants is coded as T63.

Section 24.23: OTHER/UNSPECIFIED EFFECTS OF EXTERNAL CAUSES

Other and unspecified effects of external causes is coded as T66-T78. This includes radiation sickness (T66) and effects from heat and light (T67) which includes heat syncope, heat cramps, sunstroke, and heat exhaustion. Hypothermia is coded as T68. Effects from differences in air and water pressure (T70) includes barotrauma, anoxia due to high altitude, and Caisson disease (decompression sickness).   Barotrauma are conditions that occur due to rapid changes in atmospheric pressure, such as otitis and aerosinusitis.

Note that there are many exceptions in these codes.

Asphyxiation is coded as T71 but, again, there are many exceptions. Asphyxiation can be due to plastic bags, smothered by a pillow, trapped in bed linens, smothered by another person's body, hanging or trapped in something such as a car or refrigerator.

Other deprivations are coded as T73 and include starvation, deprivation of water, and exhaustion due to excessive exertion.

Confirmed abuse and neglect of children and adults are coded as T74 including abandonment, physical or mental abuse, sexual abuse, and shaken infant syndrome. Suspected abuse is coded as T76.

Other effects from external causes include effects of lightning (T75.0), effects from vibration (T75.2), motion sickness (T75.3), and electrocution (T75.4).

Anaphylactic shock due to reaction to food is coded as T78.0. Other allergic responses such as allergic shock and anaphylaxis are coded from other T78 codes. Anaphylactic shock is the most severe type of anaphylaxis which is the body's allergic response which causes a sudden drop in the blood pressure, edema, difficulty breathing, and possibly death.

Section 24.24: EARLY COMPLICATIONS OF TRAUMA NEC

Early complications from trauma NEC are coded as T79. This includes air and fat embolism, hemorrhage, traumatic shock, anuria, ischemia and emphysema. Traumatic compartment syndrome (T79.A) occurs when there is increased pressure within an anatomic site, usually due to inflammation, that has been confined due to injury, surgery, or other medical condition.

Section 24.25: COMPLICATIONS OF MEDICAL OR SURGICAL CARE

Codes T80-T88 indicate complications of medical or surgical care with an extensive exclude note at the beginning since many of these complications are now coded under the codes for each anatomic system.   These codes include complications following infusion, transfusions and injections (T80). Air embolisms following infusions, transfusions and injections are coded as T80.0 and infections as T80.2. Blood and Rh incompatibility are coded as T80.3.

Postprocedural shock is coded as T81.1. Disruption of wounds are coded as T81.3. Infection following a procedure is coded as T81.4. A foreign body left in the body after a procedure is coded as T81.5. T81.51 are for adhesion complications. Other complications from foreign bodies left in the body include perforation and obstruction. T82-T85 are for complications due to mechanical devices and implants, e.g. displacement of breast prosthesis and implant (T85.42).

INJURIES QUIZ 18

1) What are the codes for a patient who is diagnosed with pneumothorax due to gunshot wound?

2) What are the codes for a patient who is diagnosed with a laceration of the right patella with dislocation?

3) What are the codes for a patient who is diagnosed with a third degree burn of the chest area?

4) What are the codes for a patient who is diagnosed with comminuted fracture of the shaft of the left humerus with dislocation?

5) What are the codes for a patient who is diagnosed with pneumothorax due to stab wound in the chest?

6) What are the codes for a patient who is diagnosed with swelling of right thumb due to a non-venomous spider bite?

7) What are the codes for a patient who is diagnosed with a sprain of the lateral medial collateral ligament of the right knee?

8) What are the codes for a patient who is diagnosed with swelling and fever due to rattlesnake bite on her right ankle?

9) What are the codes for a patient who is diagnosed with second degree burns of the upper right arm?

10) What are the codes for a patient who is diagnosed with a pathological fracture of the femur?

11) What are the codes for a patient who is diagnosed with frostbite with necrosis of the right ear?

12) What are the codes for a patient who is diagnosed with a sprain of the posterior cruciate ligament of the left knee?

13) What are the codes for a patient who is diagnosed with crushing injury of the left lower leg and foot?

14) What are the codes for a small child who was seen for a bean in his right ear?

CHAPTER 25
ICD-10 EXTERNAL CAUSE CODES

You will learn the following objectives in this chapter:

A. Alphabetical Index
B. Transport Accident
C. Accidents
D. Exposure to Inanimate Mechanical Devices
E. Exposure to Animate Mechanical Devices
F. Nontransport Drowning
G. Exposure to Electrical Current/Radiation
H. Exposure to Fire/Hot Substances
I. Exposure to Forces of Nature
J. Harm
K. Medical Complications
L. Supplementary Factors

Chapter 20 are the former E codes and are described as "External Causes of Morbidity" and ranges from V00-Y99. As previously noted, poisoning and adverse effects from substances are no longer included in these codes but are coded in the previously discussed injury section. E codes answer the questions, how, why and where an injury or condition occurred. External causes (E codes) include codes for "environmental events, circumstances, and conditions as the cause of injury, poisoning, and other adverse effects".

Section 25.1: ALPHABETICAL INDEX

External cause codes are not found in the Alphabetical Index for the regular codes but rather have their own alphabetical index which follows the Drugs and Chemical Table.

Section 25.2: TRANSPORT ACCIDENT

Transport accident codes include V00-V99. Definitions of all types of transport vehicles are provided in this section.

Transport accident is "any accident involving a device designed primarily for, or being used at the time primarily for, conveying persons or goods from one place to another".

Farm and construction machines are considered to be machinery unless they were on a highway and used for transportation, not work.

A device which can travel by more than one means, such as water and highways, is coded with regards to where it was being used at the time of the accident, so if it was being used on a highway then it is considered a motor vehicle.

When people are injured by a transport device that is being used for purposes other than transportation, then it would not be coded as a transport accident, such as maintenance work, other injuries unrelated to transport (such as a fight on a plane), industrial work, and sports when the device was not involved in the injury.

Pedestrians injured by a transport device are coded as V00 which includes roller-skating, skateboarding, scooter, ice skates, sleds, snowboarding, skiing, wheelchair, and baby stroller. Injuries sustained by a pedestrian by a pedal bicycle are coded as V01. Pedestrian injury caused by a two- or three-wheeled motor vehicle are coded as V02 which includes various modes of transportation by the pedestrian at the time such as walking, roller skates and skateboarding.

Pedestrian injured in a collision with a car, truck or van is coded as V03 with reference to pedestrian's mode of transportation such as walking, roller skates or skateboarding.

Pedestrian injured in collision with a train is coded as V05. Pedestrian injured in collision with other non-motor vehicle such as animal-drawn vehicle is coded as V06.

Injuries sustained by a person on a pedal bicycle is similar to the pedestrian codes as differentiated by what object the bicyclist collided with (V10-V19). Motorcycle riders sustaining injuries are differentiated by what object the rider collided with such as animal or car (V20-V29).

Injuries sustained by an occupant (driver or passenger) in a three-wheeled motor vehicle are differentiated in the same manner as the previous codes as to what it collided with (V30-V39). Codes for occupants in a car, truck or van are coded in the same manner according to what the car collided with (V40-V59). If the vehicle is a heavy transport vehicle, then the codes are V60-V69. Occupants of buses involved in an accident are coded in the same manner (V70-V79). Other means of transport are coded as V80-V89 and include animal-riders, train, streetcar, industrial vehicle, agricultural vehicle, and off-road vehicles.

Injuries sustained during an accident involving a water transport vehicle (V90-V94) include drowning, crushing, burn, falling, struck, and submersion while on various vehicles such as a boat or ship. Injuries sustained from an accident involving an air and space transport vehicle (V95-V97) include helicopters, gliders, private or commercial planes, and spacecraft.

Section 25.3: ACCIDENTS

Accidental falls, tripping, slipping, and stumbling (W00-S19) are classified by how the patient fell, such as from stairs or ladder, if it was from one level to another or not, and if there were other factors involved. This includes falls due to icy conditions or from objects such as chairs, bed, tree, cliff, and playground equipment. Codes are also differentiated by falls into certain places such as a swimming pool, well, dock, and bathtub. These codes are much more detailed than they were in the ICD-9 codes.

Section 25.4: EXPOSURE TO INANIMATE MECHANICAL FORCES

Exposure to inanimate mechanical forces (W20-W49) include being struck or thrown from an object such as piece of machinery or sports equipment. Being caught, crushed or jammed between objects is coded as W23.

Injuries sustained by contact with glass is coded as W25. Contact with tools is differentiated by whether they are powered or not (W27). Injuries caused by accidental discharge of guns is coded as W32 to w33.

Injuries caused by explosions (W35-W40) can be caused by rupture of a boiler or pressurized pipe or hose. It can also occur due to fireworks, blasting materials and explosive gases. Exposure to loud noises are coded as W42.

Foreign body or object entering through the skin is coded as W45 and is differentiated by what the foreign body or object was, such as paper or nail. Contact with needles is coded as W46.

Section 25.5: EXPOSURE TO ANIMATE MECHANICAL FORCES

Exposure to animate mechanical forces (W50-W64) include being hit, struck, kicked, bitten, twisted, scratched, crushed, pushed, or stepped on by another person. Contact with rodents is coded as W53 including mice, rats, and squirrels. Being bitten or struck by a dog is coded as W54. Contact with other animals (W55) include cats, horses, cows, and pigs. Contact with marine animals (W56) includes dolphins, whales, or sharks. Contact with crocodiles or alligators is coded as W58. Contact with nonvenomous reptiles is coded as W59. Contact with birds is coded as W61.

Section 25.6: NON-TRANSPORT DROWNING

Non-transport drownings (W65-W74) include while in bath-tub, pool, or lake.

Section 25.7: EXPOSURE TO ELECTRICAL CURRENT/RADIATION

Exposure to electrical current, radiation and extreme ambient air temperature and pressure (W85-W99) include exposure to electric transmission lines or current, radiation, UV light, lasers, excessive cold or heat, and excessive air pressure changes.

Section 25.8: EXPOSURE TO FIRE/HOT SUBSTANCES

Accidents due to fire and flames (X00-X08) include fires, smoke, explosion, fumes, and burns occurring in different types of structures and on clothing. Contact with heat and hot substances (X10-X19) include hot drinks, fats, water, gases, appliances, tools, and metals.

Section 25.9: EXPOSURE TO FORCES OF NATURE

Exposure to forces of nature (X30-X39) include cold, sunlight, earthquake, volcanoes, hurricanes, blizzards, dust storms, tidal waves, and floods. Exposures to other specified factors (X52, X58) include being in a weightless environment.

Section 25.10: HARM

Various types of harm by various means include intentional self-harm (X71-X83), assault by someone else (X92-Y08), terrorism, wars and military operations (Y35-Y38). These codes have been greatly expanded to include many reasons and involvement within these codes.

Section 25.11: MEDICAL COMPLICATIONS

Complications due to medical and surgical care that are not coded elsewhere are coded as Y62 to Y84. Misadventures to patients during surgical and medical care (Y62-Y69) include failure to properly sterilize, wrong dosage of drugs, contaminated medical substances, and non-administration of surgical and medical care. Complications with medical devices (Y70-Y82) include devices involved with anesthetic, cardiovascular, otorhinolaryngological, gastroenterology, neurological, obstetric, gynecological, ophthalmic, radiological, and orthopedic procedures. Abnormal reactions by patients to healthcare (Y83-Y84) include responses that did not occur at the time of the procedure and include amputation and removal of organs or body parts, cardiac catheterization, dialysis, radiological, and aspiration of fluids.

Section 25.12: SUPPLEMENTARY FACTORS

Supplementary factors related to cause of morbidity classified elsewhere (Y90-Y99) include blood alcohol level (Y90), place of occurrence (Y92), activity codes (Y93) which include swimming, ice skating, climbing, and baseball. External cause status (Y99) include status as a civilian, military, or volunteer.

LATE EFFECTS/POISONINGS QUIZ 19

1) What is the code for a patient with an embolism due to their pacemaker?

2) What is the code for a patient with gastritis after ingesting Percodan with alcohol and OTC antihistamines?

3) What is the code for a patient with scar tissue due to a second and third degree burn on both legs six months ago?

4) What is the code for a patient with dislocation of an artificial hip joint?

5) What is the code for a patient with CMV infection due to transplanted liver?

6) What is the code for a patient with joint pain of the knees from rickets a year ago?

7) What is the code for a patient with a pressure ulcer with necrosis from her cast of the left lower leg due to a fractured upper tibia?

8) What is the code for a patient with esophageal reflux due to ingestion of drain cleaner as an attempted suicide?

9) What is the code for a patient with failure of skin graft of the left upper arm sustained after a burn six months ago when boiling water fell on her?

10) What is the code for a right-handed patient with hemiparesis of the left side due to a CVA four months ago?

11) What is the code for a patient with mental retardation due to viral encephalitis more than 5 years ago?

12) What is the code for a patient with ataxia due to alcohol and carbamazepine?

13) What is the code for a patient with an infection and pain due to his peritoneal dialysis catheter?

14) What is the code for a patient with sequelae from a gunshot wound of the right leg a month ago?

15) What is the code for a patient with dihescence of a mastectomy wound a week ago with infection?

CHAPTER 26
FACTORS INFLUENCING HEALTH STATUS AND CONTACT

You will learn the following objectives in this chapter:

- A. Medical Necessity
- B. Sequencing
- C. Alphabetical Index
- D. Examinations
- E. Retained Foreign Body
- F. Communicable Diseases
- G. Reproduction
  1. Contraception
  2. Procreative
  3. Pregnancy
  4. Outcome of Delivery
  5. Liveborn
- H. Prophylactic Care
- I. Artificial Openings
- J. Aftercare
- K. Donors
- L. Procedures Not Completed
- M. Living Conditions
- N. Blood Type
- O. Body Mass
- P. Other Circumstances
- Q. History
- R. Status
- S. Dependence on Machines

Chapter 21 are the former V codes and are described as "Factors Influencing Health Status and Contact with the Health Services" and range from Z00-Z99. There are three conditions under which a V code may be applied:
(1) When a person who is not currently sick encounters the health services for some specific purposes.
(2) When a person with a known disease or injury, whether it is current or resolving, encounters the health care system for a specific treatment of that disease or injury.
(3) When some circumstance or problem is present which influences the person's health status but is not in itself a current illness or injury.

Section 26.1: MEDICAL NECESSITY

Because of the nature of the Z codes, they provide ICD-10 documentation of the necessity of services provided either because there is no documented diagnosis or symptom which can be coded or as supplementation to other codes to ensure that reimbursement will be provided.

Section 26.2: SEQUENCING

Most Z codes are secondary codes and should be listed second to the codes for the diagnosis or symptoms. There are some exceptions, however, when Z codes would be listed first. These exceptions are based on when the Z code describes the main reason for the healthcare visit, such as therapy codes. For example, a patient may have carcinoma and is being seen for chemotherapy. The coding guidelines in the front of the coding book outlines these issues of sequencing.

Section 26.3: ALPHABETICAL INDEX

Finding the Z codes in the alphabetical index can be challenging because they are listed under a large number of general terms including:

Admission	Exposure
Aftercare	Family history
Attention to	Fitting
Boarder	Follow-up
Care	Maintenance
Carrier	Maladjustment
Checking	Observation
Contact	Personal history
Contraception	Problem
Convalescence	Prophylactic
Counseling	Replacement
Delivery outcome	Screening
Dependence	Status
Donor	Supervision
Encounter	Transplant
Examination	

For this reason, it is recommended that you familiarize yourself with the contents of the Z code section to see what types of categories are listed. If you are familiar with the sections you will be able to find codes in the tabular Z listings rather than in the alphabetical index.

Section 26.4: EXAMINATIONS

Patients are seen by healthcare providers for a wide variety of examinations which are coded as Z00-Z13. Z00 is for visits in which the patient had no complaint or suspected diagnosis. Z00.0 is for a general adult exam, otherwise known as a well check.

A well check for a child is also now included in this same area of codes which is Z00.1 and is differentiated by age of the child. Newborns are up to 28 days and are coded as Z00.11-. For older children codes Z00.12 are used who are over 28 days of age. One code is used to indicate abnormal findings and another indicates without abnormal findings. Visit for a child experiencing rapid growth is coded as Z00.2. Delayed growth is coded as Z00.7 codes.

Examination and encounters for someone who may be a possible donor is coded as Z00.5. Exams for other reasons, such as for vision, hearing, dental, and blood pressure are coded with Z01 codes. Gynecological exams are coded as Z01.4 including a PAP test. Encounters to test patients prior to a surgical procedure (pre-procedural) are coded as Z01.8. Encounters for other reasons, such as admission to schools, armed forces, jobs, paternity testing, and blood-alcohol levels are coded with Z02 codes.

Encounters for observation are coded as Z03. Encounters for suspected maternal and fetal conditions that are eventually ruled out after testing and examination are coded with Z03 codes.

Examinations and encounters following transports or work accidents are coded with Z04 codes as well as for alleged rape, alleged physical abuse, and psychiatric evaluation.

Follow-up codes are now described as "Encounter for follow-up examination after completed treatment for malignant neoplasm" which is much clearer than it was in the ICD-9 codes. Codes Z08 are for follow-up after completed treatment for neoplasm. For follow-up of other conditions that are not related to neoplasm, code Z09 should be used.

Exams and encounters for screening for infectious and parasitic diseases are coded with codes Z11. Encounters for screening for malignant neoplasms are coded with codes Z12. Encounters for screening of other diseases (Z13) include blood disorders, diabetes mellitus, developmental disorders, metabolic, genetic, eyes and ears, cardiovascular, and other anatomic sites.

Genetic carriers and genetic susceptibility to diseases (Z14-Z15) include hemophilia A (asymptomatic or symptomatic), and cystic fibrosis.

Resistance to antimicrobial drugs (Z16) include resistance to antibiotics which are specifically listed by drug name, and antimicrobial drugs.

Estrogen receptor status (Z17) is differentiated as to negative or positive status.

Section 26.5: RETAINED FOREIGN BODY

The presence of a foreign body can be coded from various sections including S and T. However, if a foreign body remains in the body it is coded as Z18. This can include fragments that are radioactive, metal, plastic, organic such as a tooth or wood or other such as glass or stones.

Section 26.6: COMMUNICABLE DISEASES

If a person has been exposed and it has been confirmed that the organism is present in their system but they are not exhibiting symptoms, then they are carriers or suspected carriers. Patients with potential health hazards related to communicable diseases (Z20-Z28) include contact and possible exposure to communicable diseases is coded by anatomic site or type such as intestinal infectious diseases (Z20.0) and rabies (Z20.3).

Patients diagnosed as being asymptomatic with HIV are coded as Z21. HIV positive NOS is also included in these codes. B20 is used if the patient tested positive for the virus and has displayed symptoms related to it, otherwise known as AIDS which is the disease process. Z21 indicates that the patient tested positive but has not displayed any symptoms related to HIV and, therefore, does not have AIDS.

If a patient seeks healthcare to receive vaccinations or inoculations, then these are coded as Z23. These can be for single vaccinations or combinations. If they are provided during a well check for a child, the well check should be listed first.

If immunizations are not completed which can be for a variety of reasons, it would be coded with Z28 codes. Reasons for immunizations not being done or patient not receiving a full regimen for a vaccination include when it is contraindicated due to illness in the patient, allergic reaction, patient refusal, patient had the disease, or patient not returning.

Section 26.7: REPRODUCTION

Codes Z30 to Z39 include Persons Encountering Health Services in Circumstances Related to Reproduction and Development.

CONTRACEPTION: Contraceptive measures, such as devices, counseling, prescriptions, and surveillance of contraceptive measures are coded in this category of codes (Z30.0). Prescriptions such as for contraceptive pills, injectable and intrauterine are coded as Z30.01 codes. Counseling for instruction on their use is coded as Z30.018 and Z30.09. If a patient is being observed due to their contraception it is coded as Z30.4.

Encounter for an actual sterilization procedure is coded as Z30.2. For reversal of a sterilization procedure, code Z31 should be used.

PROCREATIVE MANAGEMENT: Procreative investigation and testing (Z31.0) includes healthcare services relating to infertility and aftercare of contraception such as reversal of sterilization. Counseling for procreation is coded as Z31.6 and Z31.8 codes.

PREGNANCY: Codes Z32 are for encounters for pregnancy testing or childbirth or childcare instruction. Z33 codes indicate if the patient is pregnant. Incidental pregnancy is coded as Z33.1 which is used when a pregnant patient is receiving medical care but the care is not related to the pregnancy such as a fracture. Two codes would need to be coded in this instance, the fracture and Z33.1.

Codes Z33.2 are used if the patient elects to terminate their pregnancy. Other codes for supervision of a normal pregnancy are Z34. These codes are divided by trimester and if this is the first pregnancy or not. The number of weeks of gestation (pregnancy) are coded as Z3A for each week from less than 10 weeks up to more than 42 weeks.

Postpartum care for the mother is coded as Z39.

OUTCOME OF DELIVERY: We discussed Z37.0 in an earlier chapter which referred to outcome of delivery when coding for the mother as the patient. This code is only used for the hospital visit for the mother in which delivery occurred to indicate the outcome of the birth and should be coded in addition to the pregnancy codes previously discussed earlier. These codes are differentiated by stillborn or liveborn and number of children. Complications of pregnancy should be coded first and outcome of delivery after.

Supervision of high risk pregnancies are now coded as O09 codes and are not included in this chapter. As a reminder, high-risk pregnancies include conditions that may increase the risk to the pregnancy, such as history of infertility, history of previous abortions, multiparity, insufficient prenatal care, and preterm labor. These codes may also include elderly primigravida (first pregnancy in a woman over 35), elderly multigravida (second or later pregnancy in an older woman over age 35), young primigravida (first pregnancy in a female less than 16 years of age), and young multigravida (second or later pregnancy in a female younger than 16 years of age).

LIVEBORN BIRTHS: Codes Z38 describe Liveborn Infants According to place of birth and type of delivery. These are codes used in the newborn's chart, not the mother's chart, in reference to the type of birth which includes a single birth or part of a multiparous birth and liveborn or stillborn. Deliveries include vaginally or cesarean. There are also codes if the baby is born outside of the hospital.

This code should always be listed FIRST and is only listed for the visit in which delivery occurred. If the newborn is transferred after birth to another hospital, even if it is on the same day, these codes would not be used at the hospital to which the newborn is transferred as delivery did not occur at the other hospital.

Section 26.8: PROPHYLACTIC CARE

Z40-Z53 codes are used to code for patients who are receiving aftercare or prophylactic care, or care to consolidate the treatment or to deal with a residual state after having previously received treatment for specific conditions. Prophylactic measures are treatments aimed at preventing a disease. Encounters for removal of parts of the body due to malignant neoplasms are coded with Z40.0 codes.

Codes for procedures performed for reasons other than remedying a health condition are coded as Z41 and include cosmetic surgery, circumcision, and ear piercing. Reconstructive and plastic surgery are coded with Z42 codes such as for breast reconstruction.

Section 26.9: ARTIFICIAL OPENINGS

Codes Z43-Z46 are for medical care provided for prosthetic devices. Codes Z43 are for various services provided for artificial openings which include tracheostomy, gastrostomy, colostomy and ileostomy. Care includes closure of openings, removal of catheter, or cleansing.

Fitting and adjustment of external prosthetic devices (Z44) can be provided for artificial arms, legs, eyes, and breast. These codes are differentiated by laterality and if the device was partial or complete.

Adjustment and management of implanted devices (Z45) include removal or replacement of implanted devices such as cardiac pacemakers, defibrillator, infusion pump, visual, hearing, VAD (vascular access device), neuropacemaker, breast implant, and myringotomies.

Fitting and adjustment of other devices (Z46) include spectacles, contact lenses, hearing aids, dental, orthodontic, and insulin pump.

Artificial opening status (Z93) indicate the presence of a surgical opening, not the actual operation to create one. Artificial openings include tracheostomy, colostomy and cystostomy.

Section 26.10: AFTERCARE

Orthopedic aftercare (Z47) are provided for removal of internal fixation devices and joint replacements.

Other postprocedural aftercare (Z48) include attention to dressings, sutures, and drains such as changing or removal.

Aftercare visits following organ transplants (Z48.2) include for heart, kidney, liver, lung or multiple organs.

Encounter for renal dialysis (Z49) is differentiated by what type of care is provided, whether preparatory or adequacy testing. ESRD (end stage renal dialysis) should also be coded (N18.6).

Encounters for antineoplastic aftercare such as radiation therapy is coded as Z51.0, Z51.1 for chemotherapy and immunotherapy, Z51.5 for palliative care and Z51.81 for therapeutic drug level monitoring.

Section 26.11: DONORS

Codes for people who donate blood are Z52.0. Skin donors are coded as Z52.1, bone as Z52.2, bone marrow as Z52.3, kidney as Z52.4, and liver as Z52.6. Donation of eggs for procreation are coded with A52.81 codes and differentiated by type of donor (anonymous or designated) and age of donor (over or under age 35). If a patient received a donated organ in the past but is not currently undergoing a procedure to implant a donated organ, this is known as status post transplanted organ and is coded as Z94.

Section 26.12: PROCEDURES NOT COMPLETED

Procedures or treatment may not be completed for various reasons (Z53) such as patient elects not to or other contraindications.

Section 26.13: LIVING CONDITIONS

Living conditions should also be reported when they may affect the management or outcome of the patient's care utilizing codes Z55-Z65. Problems related to education and literacy (Z55) include illiteracy, school failure, and discord with teachers. Problems related to employment (Z56) include unemployment, change of job, threat of job loss, stress at work, or hostile work place. Exposure to occupational risks (Z57) include noise, radiation, dust, smoke, toxic agents, extreme temperatures, and vibrations.

Problems relating to housing (Z59) include homelessness, poor surroundings, neighbor difficulties, lack of adequate food and safe drinking, poverty, loan foreclosure and creditor problems. Problems within the social environment (Z60) include empty nest syndrome, social exclusion, living alone, discrimination and migration. Problems with upbringing (Z62) include negative life events in childhood such as inadequate parental supervision or overprotection, living in foster homes, scapegoating of child, and inappropriate parental pressure. It also includes history of physical, sexual and psychological abuse. Parent-child conflict, neglect, and estrangement are also included.

Other family difficulties (Z63) include problems with spouse or partner or in-laws, military deployment or other parental absences, divorce, death of family members, alcoholism, and drugs. Psychosocial circumstances (Z64) include unwanted pregnancy, multiparity problems, problems with counselors, criminal convictions, incarceration, victim of crime, and exposure to disasters or war.

Do not resuscitate status (DNR) is coded as Z66.

Section 26.14: BLOOD TYPE

Blood types are coded as Z67 for all types, A, B, AB and O and differentiated as to Rh being negative or positive.

Section 26.15: BODY MASS

Body mass index (Z68) varies by patient's weight in kilograms for adults and percentile for children (Z68.5).

Section 26.16: OTHER CIRCUMSTANCES

Other circumstances (Z69-Z76) include encounters for mental health for child abuse (Z69.0). Abuse by spouse or partner is coded as Z69.1. For other abuse, code Z69.8 is used. Counseling related to sexual issues (Z70) include concerns about impotence, promiscuity, and sexual orientation.

Worried well is coded as Z71.1 which means the patient had good reason for concern regarding their health and so they received medical examination. Dietary counseling and surveillance is coded as Z71.3. Counseling for issues with alcohol is coded as Z71.4, for drugs as Z71.5, tobacco Z71.6, and HIV as Z71.7.

Problems related to lifestyle (Z72) include tobacco use, lack of physical exercise, inappropriate eating habits, high risk sexual behavior, gambling Z72.6, antisocial behavior as Z72.81, and problems sleeping Z72.82. Problems related to life management include burn out (Z73.0), lack of leisure (Z73.2, stress (Z73.3), different types of insomnia (Z73.81), reduced mobility (Z74.0, and need for assistance in the home (Z74.2).

Issues relating to medical facilities include patient waiting for admission to facility, unavailability of help, and holiday relief care (Z75). Malingerer (Z76.5) is someone who feigns illness.

Section 26.17: HISTORY

There are two types of histories that can be coded and are important in the provision of healthcare services which are personal and family histories (Z77-Z99). Do NOT confuse the two when selecting codes. History indicates that the condition no longer exists so do not code a personal history for a condition for which a patient is still being treated.

Histories include cancer, mental disorders, diseases, fractures, congenital malformations, allergies, surgeries, poisonings, injuries, and conditions of the circulatory, urinary, digestive, genital, skin, or other system including nutritional deficiencies. These codes also include history of drug, tobacco, or alcohol abuse and exposure to toxic substances such as asbestos and lead.

There are codes for exposure to substances (Z77) such as hazardous chemicals such as arsenic and lead, environment hazards such as mold, or bodily fluids from someone else that may be hazardous such as a person who has HIV.

Z79 codes are for long term drug therapy which are currently being taken such as anticoagulants, insulin, antibiotics, and steroids. Allergic reactions to drugs such as penicillin are coded as Z88. Food allergies are coded as Z91 for various food items, insects, latex, and radiographic dye.

Z89-Z90 indicate a person having had replacement of organ or tissue by transplant (animal or human) (status post) such as hands, legs, organs, or genitalia.

Failure to comply with medical recommendations are coded as Z91 and include noncompliance and underdosing.

History of psychological trauma (Z91.4) include abuse of adult and self-harm.

Z92 codes indicate history of use of contraceptives, drug therapy (e.g. chemotherapy and estrogen), irradiation and failed moderate sedation.

Presence of implanted devices or organs are coded as Z94-Z97 and are known as status post, meaning that the device or organ was previously implanted. These codes include cardiac grafts, heart valves, pacemakers, intraocular lens, orthopedic joint implants, and artificial eyes or limbs.

Section 26.18: STATUS

Postprocedural status (Z98) indicates that a patient received surgery in the past. This is important because it can influence decisions regarding the patient's healthcare such as intestinal bypasses, and collapsed lung.

Removal of cataracts in the past is coded as Z98.4. If patient was sterilized previously, they would be status post sterilization (Z98.5). If a patient received an angioplasty in the past it is coded as Z98.6. Breast implants are coded as Z98.82. If breast implants were removed they are coded as Z98.86.

Section 26.19: DEPENDENCE ON MACHINES

Dependence on machines while under medical care (Z99) includes aspirator, respirator, renal dialysis, wheelchair and oxygen.

SUPPLEMENTARY CODES QUIZ 20

1) What are the codes for a patient seen for follow-up exam of breast cancer which was removed a year ago and treated with chemotherapy?

2) What are the codes for a patient seen who had a replacement of their colostomy?

3) What are the codes for a patient seen today for prophylactic administration of Nolvadex for breast cancer which metastasized from skin cancer on the back which was removed a year ago with positive estrogen receptor status?

4) What are the codes for a woman who delivered a newborn who was 550 grams at 34 weeks with hyperbilirubinemia?

5) What are the codes for a patient who is leaving the country and needed a cholera vaccination?

6) What are the codes for a patient seen today for counseling regarding instructions in the use of an insulin pump for her diabetes Type I and high blood pressure?

7) What are the codes for a patient seen today for cataracts and diabetic neuropathy Type II with long term use of insulin and ASHD?

8) What are the codes for a 3-year-old child during a well check who was to receive DTP vaccination but was uncontrollable and so the vaccine was not administered?

9) What are the codes for a patient who was seen today for laparoscopic resection of the small intestine with anastomosis which had to be changed to an open procedure for cancer?

10) What are the codes for a patient seen today for routine PAP test with no findings?

11) What are the codes for a patient who is a bone marrow donor?

12) What are the codes for a patient seen today for adjustment of peritoneal dialysis catheter during dialysis?

13) What are the codes for a patient seen today for possible gout due to complaints of stomach pain but tests were negative?

14) What are the codes for a patient seen today for exercise therapy after suffering a severe crushing injury to the left lower leg four months ago?

15) What are the codes for a patient seen today for drug resistant pulmonary TB?

CHAPTER 27
ICD-10 PCS OVERVIEW PROCEDURAL CODES

You will learn the following objectives in this chapter:

- A. ICD-10 PCS Coding System
- B. Characters
    1. First Character: Section
    2. Second Character: Body System
    3. Third Character: Root Operation
    4. Fourth Character: Body Part
    5. Fifth Character: Approach
    6. Sixth Character: Device
    7. Seventh Character: Qualifier

ICD-10 Procedure Coding System (PCS) is used only for inpatient hospital procedural code and therefore, physician-based coders do not need to know this as they will be using CPT codes instead. This is a brief overview so any curious coder can gain some understanding of the coding system.

Section 27.1: ICD-10 PCS CODING SYSTEM

The goal in developing the ICD-10-PCS system is to provide completeness unique definitions, expandability, structural integrity, and is multiaxial with standardized terminology. Completeness means having unique codes for procedures that are able to expand to accommodate the growth in healthcare in procedures and services.

Section 27.2: CHARACTERS

ICD-10-PCS codes are seven characters which represent some aspect of the procedure. They are not specifically listed as one code but rather require the selection of each character one by one based on what the character represents as it relates to the procedure.

The second through seventh characters mean the same thing within each section, but may mean different things in other sections. Each character can be any of 34 possible values the ten digits 0-9 and the 24 letters A-H, J-N and P-Z may be used in each character. The letters O and I excluded to avoid confusion with the numbers 0 and 1.[2] There are no decimals in ICD-10-PCS.

Character 1 represents the section.
Character 2 represents the body system.
Character 3 represents the root operation
Character 4 represents the body part.
Character 5 represents the approach.
Character 6 represents the device.
Character 7 represents the qualifier.

For example, code 0U524ZZ is for destruction of the both ovaries which was done percutaneously with a scope but no devices or additional qualifiers were involved.

There are 16 sections in the ICD-10-PCS.

The first character represents the section which are broad such as Medical and Surgical. There are 16 sections as denoted by 0 through 9 and letters B through D and F through H.

The second character represents the body system (physiological/anatomical) such as respiratory system.

The third character represents the root operation which is the procedure or services provided.

The fourth character represents the body part which is much more specific such as the left upper leg.

The fifth character represents the approach used to gain access to the surgical site such as the procedure being open or performed with a scope.

The sixth character represents a device, if implanted although some procedures may not involve a device which would be coded with a "Z". There are four categories for devices: grafts/prosthesis, implants, simple or mechanical appliances, and electronic appliances.

The seventh character represents a qualifier which describes any special attributes of the procedure. If there is no qualifier "Z" would be used.

Section 27.3: FIRST CHARACTER

The first character represents the section which are broad such as Medical and Surgical. There are 16 sections as denoted by 0 through 9 and letters B through D and F through H.

The following is a table for the values of the first character:

SECTION VALUE	DESCRIPTION
1	Obstetrics
2	Placement
3	Administration
4	Measurement and Monitoring
5	Extracorporeal Assistance & Performance
6	Extracorporeal Therapies

7	Osteopathic
8	Other Procedures
9	Chiropractic
B	Imaging
C	Nuclear Medicine
D	Radiation Oncology
F	Physical Rehabilitation & Diagnostic Audiology
G	Mental Health
H	Substance Abuse Treatment

Placement characters are for procedures in which a device is used to protect, immobilize, stretch, compress, or pack a site.

Administration characters indicate procedures in which there is administration of a substance such as infusions, injections or transfusions.

Extracorporeal assistance refers to the use of devices to assist a patient such as mechanical ventilation.

Section 27.4: Second Character

The second character is the physiological or anatomical system where the procedure is performed. Body systems include:

VALUE	DESCRIPTION
0	Central Nervous System
1	Peripheral Nervous System
2	Heart & Great Vessels
3	Upper Arteries
4	Lower Arteries
5	Upper Veins
6	Lower Veins
7	Lymphatic & Hemic System
8	Eye

9	Ear, Nose, Sinus
B	Respiratory
C	Mouth & Throat
D	Gastrointestinal
F	Hepatobiliary & Pancreas
G	Endocrine
H	Skin & Breast
J	Subcutaneous Tissue & Fascia
K	Muscles
L	Tendons
M	Bursae & Ligaments
N	Head & Facial Bones
P	Upper Bones
Q	Lower Bones
R	Upper Joints
S	Lower Joints
T	Urinary System
U	Female Reproductive
V	Male Reproductive
W	Anatomic Region, General
X	Anatomic Regions, Upper Extremities
Y	Anatomic Regions, Lower Extremities

Section 27.5: Third Character

The third character describes the actual procedure. There are 31 different root operations. There are nine groups:

1.   Procedures that take out some/all of a body part.
2.   Procedures that take out solids/fluids/gases from a body part.

3.   Procedures involving cutting or separation only.
4.   Procedures that put in/put back or move some/all of a body part.
5.   Procedures that alter the diameter/route of a tubular body part.
6.   Procedures that always involve a device.
7.   Procedures involving examination only.
8.   Procedures defining other repairs.
9.   Procedures defining objectives.

Procedures that take out some/all of a body part include excision, resection, detachment, destruction or extraction.

Procedures that take out solids/fluids/gases from a body part include drainage, extirpation, and fragmentation.

Procedures involving cutting or separation only include division or release.

Procedures that put in/put back or move some/all of a body part include transplantation, reattachment, transfer, and repositioning.

Procedures that alter the diameter/route of a tubular body part include restriction, occlusion, dilation and bypass.

Procedures that always involve a device include insertion, replacement, supplement, change, removal and revision.

Procedures involving examination only include inspection and mapping.

Procedures defining other repairs include repair and control.

Procedures defining other repairs include fusion, alteration and creation.

Section 27.6: Fourth Character

The fourth character represents the specific anatomical site where the procedure is performed including laterality such as left lower leg.

Section 27.7: Fifth Character

The fifth character represents the approach used to get to the procedural site. Various approaches include open (0), percutaneous (3), percutaneous endoscopic (4), via natural or artificial opening (7), via natural or artificial opening endoscopic (8), via natural or artificial opening endoscopic assistance (F), and external (X).

Open involves cutting through the skin and membranes. Percutaneous means puncturing the skin or any other layer. Percutaneous endoscopic means puncturing the skin or any other layer to insert a scope. Via natural or artificial opening is an approach that uses an opening to gain access, one with a scope involved and one without. This type of approach which is also described as assistance means that additional instrumentation was inserted through the opening. External indicates that the procedure was performed on top of the skin and not cutting was involved.

Section 27.8: Sixth Character

The sixth character describes the device inserted into the body during the procedure. "Z" should be used if there is no device inserted. The types of devices are biological or synthetic material that takes the place of all or portion of body part, biological or synthetic material that assists or prevents a physiological function, therapeutic material that is not absorbed by, eliminated by, or incorporated into a body part, and mechanical or electronic appliances used to assist, monitor, take the place of or prevent a physiological function.

Values differ by procedures. Some examples include:

VALUE	DESCRIPTION
0	Drainage Device
2	Monitoring Device
3	Infusion Device
4	Internal Fixation Device
7	Autologous Tissue Substitute
8	Zooplastic Tissue
9	Autologous Venous Tissue
A	Autologous Arterial tissue
C	Extraluminal Device
D	Intraluminal Device
J	Synthetic Substitute
K	Nonautologous Tissue Substitute
L	Artificial Sphincter
M	Bone Growth Stimulator
Q	Implantable Heart Assist System
R	External Heart Assist System
T	Radioactive Intraluminal

	Device
Y	Other Device
Z	No Device

Section 27.9: Seventh Character

The seventh character provided additional information about the procedure but is not always applicable which is known as a qualifier. "Z" should be used if there is no qualifier.

Values differ by procedures. Some examples include:

VALUE	DESCRIPTION
0	Allogeneic
1	Syngeneic
2	Zoolastic
3	Monoplanar
4	Ring
5	Hybrid
6	Ureter, Right
7	Ureter, Left
8	Colon
9	Colocutaneous
A	Pacemaker Lead
B	Skin & Subcutaneous Tissue
C	Ileocutaneous
D	Cutaneous
G	Pressure Sensor
S	Biventricular
T	Ductus Arteriosus
X	Diagnostic
Z	No Qualifier

ICD-10   TEST 2

1. What is the code for a patient who is seen today for chest pains due to possible MI?

2. What is the code for a patient who is seen today for crushing chest injury?

3. What are the codes for a patient who has metastatic brain cancer?

4. What are the codes for a patient seen today for chemotherapy for ongoing treatment of breast cancer on the right side which was excised two months ago?

5. An 8-year-old patient is seen today for enteritis due to Clostridium difficile. What are the codes?

6. What are the codes for a patient who classical PKU?

7. What does HIPAA stand for?

8. What other prosecutory actions are levied besides fines for healthcare fraud?

9. What number most often represents an unspecified code?

10. What is Volume 2 of the ICD book known as?

11. Internal derangement of ligament of the left knee is what code?

12. What are the codes for a subsequent encounter for perforation of the esophagus that was traumatic?

13. What are the codes for a patient who has cancer of the anterior surface of the epiglottis?

14. What is the code for postviral encephalitis?

15. What are the two supplementary classifications in Volume 1?

16. Name and describe the three types of health record formats.

17. Describe the two types of progress notes.

18. What does CPC mean?

19. What types of coding does a CPC perform?

20. What are the codes for a patient who has obstetrical tetanus?

21. What types of coding does a CCS perform?

22. Explain the Stark Laws.

23. What are the codes for traumatic asphyxiation?

24. What are the codes for a patient who has polio due to having received the vaccine?

25. What are the codes for benign leiomyoma of the abdomen?

26. What are the codes for a patient with Reye's syndrome due to when the patient overdosed on aspirin?

27. What are the codes for an intoxicated patient who was binge drinking over the weekend and was seen in the emergency room who experienced alcoholic stupor with blood level of 42?

28. A patient is seen today for arthropathy due to TB in the left shoulder. What are the codes?

29. ICD-10-CM stands for what?

30. What federal department is CMS a part of?

31. How many volumes are there in the ICD today?

32. What are the codes for a patient seen today for septic urinary tract infection due to E. coli?

33. What are the codes for a patient seen with hepatitis D associated with inactive Hepatitis B?

34. What are the codes for a 42-year-old patient who has ASHD in the right leg with gangrene and an ulcer with necrosis where a nonautologous bypass graft was previously inserted?

35. What are the codes for a patient with uveitis due to syphilis?

36. What is the code for a patient with acute and subacute bronchitis due to Pseudomonas

37. What are the codes for malaria with pernicious complications with hepatitis?

38. What are the codes for a patient who has encephalitis from a tick bite?

39. What are the codes for a patient who has arthritis of the left hand due to staph infection?.

40. What are the codes for a 23-year-old patient who is seen today for MRSA?

41. What are the codes for leiomyoma of the uterus?

42. What are the codes for a patient who is seen today for nausea and vomiting due to chemotherapy?

43. What are the codes for a patient with carcinoma of the breast metastatic to the left lung?

44. AHIMA stands for what?

45. What does CCS-P mean?

46. What are the codes for patient experiencing panic attack with agoraphobia?

47. What are the codes for a patient who has MS?

48. What are the codes for a patient who has pars planitis?

49. What are the codes for a patient who is experiencing combat fatigue?

50. What are the codes for a left snapping knee?

51. A patient is seen today for a stomach ache and headache and was found to be due to pathogenic E. coli food poisoning. What are the codes?

52. What age is typically defined as presenile dementia?

53. What are the codes for a patient with anorexia?

54. What are the codes for a patient who has dermatitis due to contact with chromium?

55. What are the codes for a patient suffering from depression and grief due to the death of her husband?

56. Describe the CNS.

57. What are the codes for a patient who has juvenile scoliosis in the cervicothoracic area of unknown cause?

58. What are the codes for a patient with a classic migraine that is not responding to treatment?

59. What are the codes for a patient who has spina bifida occulta?

60. What are the codes for a patient who has meningitis due to Aerobacter aerogenes?

61. What are the codes for a patient who has double vision?

62. What is the difference between hemiplegia and hemiparesis?

63. Infantile cerebral palsy occurs when?

64. What are the codes for a patient who has Fusarium keratitis?

65. What are the codes for a patient who has moderate malnutrition due to low intake of protein?

66. What are the codes for a patient who has osteitis with chronic mastoiditis due to TB?

67. What does idiopathic mean?

68. When two major changes were added in the ninth revision?

69. What are the codes for septicemia due to anthrax?

70. What are the codes for a patient who has erythema multiforme major with inflammation of the eyelid?

71. What are the codes for a pregnant patient who has pneumonia due to anesthesia with aspiration?

72. What are the codes for a patient who has Huntington's dementia?

73. What are the codes for perforation of the esophagus?

74. What is the difference between a TIA and a CVA?

75. What are the fines for healthcare fraud?

APPENDIX A
COMBINING FORMS & ABBREVIATIONS

A

a, an	absence, without
ab	away from
abdomino	abdomen
ac	pertaining to
acous	hearing
acro	extremity
acusis	hearing
ad	toward
adeno	gland
adip	fatty
adren	adrenal glands
emia	blood condition
al	pertaining to
abl	white
algia	pain
allo	different
ambi	two
an	not, without
angio	blood vessel
ante	before
anti	against
arthro	joints
aur	ear
auto	self
axill	armpit

B

bi	two
bio	life
blepharo	eyelid
brachio	arm
brady	slow
bucco	cheek

C

capit	head
carcin	cancer
cardio	heart
carp	wrist
cele	hernia, pouch
centesis	surgical puncture

(continued)

cephal	head
cerebr	brain
cervic	neck
cholecysto	gall bladder
chrondro	cartilage
circum	around
contra	against
costo	rib
crine	secrete
cryo	cold
cutan	skin
cyano	blue color
cyst	urinary bladder
cyt	cell

D

dactyl	finger, toe
de	away from
dermato	skin
dia	through
dis	take apart
dorso	back
dynia	pain
dys	bad

E

ec	out, away
ectasis	dilation
ectomy	excision
emesis	vomiting
emia	blood condition
endo	within
entero	intestine
eu	good
ex	out

G

gastro	stomach
gen	to form
genu	knee
gingiv	gums
gloss	tongue

gluco	sugar, glucose	meso	middle
glycol	sugar	meta	change
gram	record, picture	micro	small
graph	record, picture	mono	single
graphy	process of recording	morpho	form, shape
		myo	muscle
		myelo	bone marrow
H		myringo	eardrum
hemato	blood	myxo	mucus
hemi	one-half		
hepato	liver		
hetero	other	**N**	
histo	tissue	necro	death
hydro	water	neo	new
hyper	above	nephro	kidney
hypo	below	neuro	nerve
hysteron	uterus		
		O	
I		oculo	eye
ia	condition	odon	teeth
iatro	medicine, treatment	odyn	pain
idio	self	oid	resembling
infra	below	oligo	few, little
inter	between	oma	tumor
intra	within	omphalo	navel
ism	condition	onco	tumor
iso	equal	onycho	nail
ist	one who specializes	ophthalmo	eye
it is	inflammation	oro	mouth
ium	tissue, structure	ortho	straight
		ose	full
K		osis	abnormal condition
kerato	cornea	osteo	bone
		oto	ear
L			
labio	lip	**P**	
lacrimo	tear	palpebro	eyelid
laparo	abdomen	pan	all
lingu	tongue	para	abnormal
lipo	fat	paresis	paralysis
litho	stone, calculus	patho	disease
logo	knowledge	ped	foot
lysis	destruction	penia	deficiency
		pepsia	digestion
M		per	through
macro	large	peri	surrounding
malacia	softening	pexy	fixation
megaly	enlargement	phage	eating
melano	black	pharmaco	drug

pharyng	pharynx	sangui	blood
phlebo	veins	sarco	flesh
phobo	fear	scope	instrument for viewing
phono	sound	semi	half
photo	light	sialo	saliva
phren	diaphragm	sinistro	left
plasia	formation	sis	condition
plasty	surgical repair	somato	body
plegia	paralysis	splen	spleen
pleura	ribs	spondylo	vertebrae
pneumo	lungs	stasis	stop
pod	foot	steno	narrowing
poiesis	production	stoma	mouth
poly	many	stomy	creation of an opening
post	after	sub	underneath
pre	before	super	above, excess
presbyo	old	supra	above
pro	before	syn	together, with
procto	rectum		
psycho	mind	**T**	
ptosis	drooping, falling	tachy	fast
ptysis	spitting	thoraco	chest
pulmon	lungs	thrombo	blood clot
pyo	pus	toco	childbirth
pyro	fever	tome	cutting instrument
		tomy	cutting
R		trans	across
rachio	spine	tripsy	crushing
re	back	trophy	development
ren	kidney	tympano	eardrum
retro	back		
rhino	nose	**U**	
rrhage	burst forth	ule	small
rrhaphy	suture	ultra	beyond, excessive
rrhea	flow, discharge	ungui	nail
		uni	one
S			

APPENDIX B
ABBREVIATIONS

AB	abortion
AD	right ear
ADD	attention deficit disorder
AIDS	acquired immune Deficiency syndrome
ALS	amyotrophic lateral Sclerosis
AMA	against medical advice
AP	anteroposterior
AS	left ear
AU	both ears
BBB	bundle branch block
BKA	below knee amputation
BPH	benign prostatic hyperplasia
Bx	biopsy
CA	cancer
CABG	coronary artery bypass graft
CAD	coronary artery disease
CAPD	continuous ambulatory Peritoneal dialysis
CAT	computerized axial tomography
CBC	complete blood count
CC	chief complaint
CHD	coronary heart disease
CHF	congestive heart failure
CNS	central nervous system
COPD	chronic obstructive pulmonary disease
CRF	chronic renal failure
C-section	cesarean section
CSF	cerebrospinal fluid
CT	computed tomography
CVA	cerebrovascular accident
CX	chest x-ray
D&C	dilation and curettage
DM	diabetes mellitus

DNR	do not resuscitate
DT	delirium tremens
DTR	deep tendon reflexes
Dx	diagnosis
EEG	electroencephalogram
EENT	eyes, ears, nose and throat
EGD	esophagogastroduodenoscopy
EKG	electrocardiogram
ESRD	end stage renal disease
ESWL	extracorporeal shock wave Lithotripsy
Fx	fracture
G	gravid (pregnancy)
GERD	gastroesophageal reflux Disease
HIPAA	Health Insurance Portability& Accountability Act
HIV	human immunodeficiency virus
HPI	History of present illness
HTN	hypertension
IBD	irritable bowel disease
I&D	incision and drainage
IHD	ischemic heart disease
IOL	intraocular lens
IPPB	intermittent positive pressure Breathing
IVP	intravenous pyelogram
KUB	kidney, ureter & bladder x-ray
LA	left atrium
LAD	left anterior descending coronary Artery

Lat	lateral	p.o.	by mouth
LBBB	left bundle branch block	prn	as needed
LFT	liver function test	PSA	prostate specific antigen
LLL	left lower lobe (lung)	PTCA	percutaneous transluminal Coronary angioplasty
LP	lumbar puncture		
LVAD	left ventricular assist device	PTH	parathyroid hormone
		PTSD	post traumatic stress disorder
MAC	monitored anesthesia care		
MMR	measles, mumps, rubella	PVC	premature ventricular contraction
MRI	magnetic resonance imaging		
		RA	rheumatoid arthritis
		RBBB	right bundle branch block
NB	newborn	RBC	red blood count
NICU	neonatal intensive care unit	RDS	respiratory distress syndrome
NSAID	nonsteroidal anti-inflammatory Drug		
		R/O	rule out
		SC	subcutaneous
OA	osteoarthritis	SARS	severe acute respiratory syndrome
OB/GYN	obstetrics/gynecology		
OD	right eye	SIDS	sudden infant death syndrome
ORIF	open reduction internal fixation		
		SLE	systemic lupus erythematosus
PA	posteroanterior	SOAP	subjective, objective, assessment, plan
PAC	premature atrial contraction		
Para	number of viable births	SOB	short of breath
PD	peritoneal dialysis	SVC	superior vena cava
PEEP	positive end-expiratory pressure	SVD	spontaneous vaginal delivery
PEG	percutaneous endoscopic Gastrostomy (feeding tube)	T&A	tonsillectomy and adenoidectomy
PERRLA	pupils equal, round and reactive To light and accommodation	TAB	therapeutic abortion
		TAH	total abdominal hysterectomy
PET	positive emission tomography	TB	tuberculosis
		TIA	transient ischemic attack
PE tube	ventilating tube for eardrum	TM	tympanic membrane
		TNM	tumor, nodes, metastases
PID	pelvic inflammatory disease	TPN	total parenteral nutrition
PIP	proximal interphalangeal joint	TVH	total vaginal hysterectomy
PKU	phenylketonuria	UA	urinalysis
PMH	past medical history	URI	upper respiratory infection
PMS	premenstrual syndrome	UTI	urinary tract infection

APPENDIX C
RESOURCES

Medical Coding Specialist's Exam Review, Lyn Olsen, 2006, Cengage/Delmar Publishing Co.

Correct Coding for Medicare, Compliance, and Reimbursement, Belinda Frisch, 2007, Cengage/Delmar Publishing.

Today's Health Information Management, Dana McWay, Thomson/Delmar, 2008.

International Classification of Diseases-9th Revision-Clinical Modification, 2013.

Current Procedural Terminology, American Medical Association, 2009.

Healthcare Common Procedure Coding System, CMS, 2009.

CPT: Beyond the Basics. Gail Smith. AHIMA, 2000.

Netter's Atlas of Human Anatomy for CPT Coding. Celeste Kirschner, AMA, 2005.

The Complete Procedure Coding Book. Shelley Safian, McGraw-Hill, 2009.

Centers for Medicare and Medicaid Services, Health and Human Services, www.cms.hhs.gov

National Center for Healthcare Statistics, www.cdc.gov/nchs/

"ICD-10: Coding Fundamentals", M. Sue Meads & Faye Brown, PMIC, 1999.

"ICD-10-CM, ICD-10-PCS Preview," Anita Hazelwood & Carol Venable, AHIMA, 2004.

ICD-10-CM Complete Draft Code Set, 2014.

STRUCTURE QUIZ 1

1. What number most often represents an unspecified code? 9

2. What is the code for encephalopathy that is not specified? G93.40

3. Derangement of a previous ligament of the right knee is what code? M23.8X1

4. What are the codes for a perforation of the esophagus that was traumatic? S27.819A

5. What number most often represents a code in which more information is provided but there is no specific code for the condition? 8

6. What is the code for spina bifida occulta?   Q76.0

7. What are the codes for otitis due to impetigo? L01.00

8. What are the codes for excessive vomiting in a pregnant woman? O21.9

9. What does NEC stand for? Not elsewhere classified

10. What is the code for postviral encephalitis? B97.89

11. What is the code for a patient who is seen today for crushing chest injury? S27.9XXA

12. A patient is seen today for a headache and polyneuropathy due to Type 1 diabetes. What are the codes? E10.40, R51

13. A patient is seen today to rule out a hernia due to abdominal pain. What are the codes? R51

14. A patient is seen today for arthropathy due to TB of the hip. What are the codes? A18.02

15. A patient is seen today for a stomach ache and headache and was found to be due to botulism. What are the codes? A05.1

INFECTIOUS DISEASES QUIZ 2

1. Is AIDS pandemic or epidemic? pandemic

2. What are the codes for septicemia due to anthrax? A22.7

3. What are the codes for a patient seen today for septic urinary tract infection due to E. coli? N39.0, B96.20,, A41.9

4. What are the codes for a patient seen with hepatitis D associated with Hepatitis B? B17.0

5. What are the codes for a patient with uveitis due to syphilis? A51.43

6. What are the codes for a patient who has H. influenza due to meningitis? G00.0

7. What are the codes for a patient who has infection of the colon due to Clostridium difficile? A04.7

8. What are the codes for a patient seen today for HIV and related Kaposi's sarcoma of the lymph nodes? B20, G46.3

9. What are the codes for a patient seen today with HIV? Z21

10. What are the codes for chronic spondylitis? M46.90

11. What are the codes for a patient seen today for bacteremia with septic shock? R78.81 R65.21

12. What are the codes for a patient with acute bronchitis due to Pseudomonas? J21.8, B96.5

13. What are the codes for a patient with pernicious complications with nephropathy? B52.0

14. What are the codes for a patient seen today for SIRS with septic shock? R65.21

15. What are the codes for a 23-year-old patient who is seen today for MRSA? B95.62

NEOPLASMS QUIZ 3

1. What are the codes for intramural leiomyoma of the uterus? D25.1

2. What are the codes for a patient who is seen today for nausea and vomiting due to chemotherapy two days ago? R11.2, C80.1, T45.1X5

3. What are the codes for traumatic asphyxiation? S27.9XX

4. What are the codes for benign leiomyoma of the abdomen? D21.4

5. What are the codes for a patient who has metastatic brain cancer? C79.31

6. What are the codes for Paget's disease of the extramammary skin? C44.90

7. What are the codes for a patient with carcinoma of the body of the uterus and contiguous sites? C54.8

8. What are the codes for carcinoma of the rectum and colon metastatic from the anterior wall of the bladder? C67.3, C78.5

9. What are the codes for adenoma of the chief cell? D35.1

10. What are the codes for a patient who is seen today for prophylactic chemotherapy a year after having a mastectomy due to breast cancer with treatment completed three months ago? Z41.8, Z85.01

11. What are the codes for a patient who has Hodgkin's lymphoma of the lymph nodes of the neck and axilla and the spleen? C81.98, C81.97

12. What are the codes for patient with malignant schwannoma of the abdomen? C49.4

13. What are the codes for leiomyoblastoma (include the M code) of the chest? D48.1

14. What are the codes for osteochondroma of the coccyx? D16.8

15. What are the codes for patient with UTI due to E. coli? N39.0, B96.20

BLOOD DISORDERS QUIZ 4

1. What are the codes for a patient with senile dementia? F03.90

2. What are the codes for a patient experiencing septic shock due to UTI? N39.0, R65.21303

3. What are the codes for a patient suffering from dipsomania? F10.20

4. What are the codes for a patient with goat's milk anemia? D52.8

5. What are the codes for a patient who metastatic cancer of the uterus? C79.82

6. What are the codes for an anemic patient due to hemorrhaging of a lower leg wound caused by a car accident? S81.829A, D62, V49.9XXA

7. What are the codes for a patient who has sickle cell anemia Hb-SS with acute chest syndrome? D57.00, J99

8. What are the codes for a patient who has vegan anemia? D518

9. What are the codes for a patient who has malignant schwannoma of the hip? C49.20

10. What are the codes for a patient experiencing a crisis with sickle cell anemia? D57.00

11. What are the codes for a patient who is diagnosed with anemia due to a chronic gastric ulcer? K25.7, D63.8

12. What are the codes for a patient with Hodgkins lymphoma of the spleen and axillary and neck lymph nodes who has neutropenia due to chemotherapy? C81.97, C81.98, D7.01

13. What are the codes for a patient with traumatic asphyxiation? S27.9XXA

14. What are the codes for a patient with a coagulation defect due to Vitamin K deficiency? D68.4

15. What are the codes for a patient who Pelger-Huet anomaly? D72.0

ENDOCRINE QUIZ 5

1. What are the codes for a patient with drug-induced Cushing's syndrome? E24.2

2. What are the codes for a patient with H. influenza with meningitis? G00.0

3. What are the codes for a patient with anemia and ALS? G12.21, D64.9

4. What are the codes for a patient with polyuria due to possible diabetes mellitus? R35.8

5. What are the codes for a Type I diabetic patient with cataracts? E10.9, H26.9

6. What are the codes for a patient with arthritis due to chronic gout? M1A.9XX0

7. What are the codes for a patient with Hodgkins lymphoma of the spleen and axillary and neck lymph nodes? C81.97, C81.98

8. What are the codes for a patient treated with insulin in the emergency room due to severe ketoacidosis due to their diabetes mellitus? E11.69

9. What are the codes for a patient who experienced hypovolemic shock due to trauma? T79.4XXA

10. What are the codes for a patient with goiter related to hyperthyroidism with storm? E05.01

11. What are the codes for a patient with diabetic retinal microangiopathy with edema? E11.311

12. What are the codes for a patient with a headache and possible concussion? R51

13. What are the codes for hypopituitarism due to the administration of radiotherapy? E23.1, T66.XXXA

14. What are the codes for a patient experiencing a thyrotoxic crisis due to Graves' Disease? E05.01

15. What are the codes for a patient who has amputation of two toes on the right foot due to gangrene related to Type 2 diabetic peripheral vascular disease? E11.52

MENTAL QUIZ 6

1. What are the codes for a patient with carcinoma of the lower outer quadrant of the breast metastatic to the left lung?   C50.519, C78.02

2. What are the codes for patient experiencing panic attack with agoraphobia? F40.01

3. What are the codes for a patient who is experiencing combat fatigue? F430

4. What are the codes for a patient who has chronic alcoholism with cirrhosis? F10.20, K70.30

5. What are the codes for a patient with anorexia? R63.0

6. What are the codes for a patient suffering from depression due to the death of her husband? F43.21

7. What are the codes for a teenager who has been experiencing problems with significant school truancy? F91.2

8. What are the codes for a patient with subacute borderline schizophrenia? F20.89

9. What are the codes for a patient with a long history of alcoholism who was binge drinking over the superbowl weekend and seen for drunkenness? F10.229

10. What are the codes for a patient with dementia due to alcohol intoxication? F10.27

11. What are the codes for a 62-year-old patient with paranoid senile dementia? F03.90

12. What are the codes for a patient with bulima nervosa? F50.2

13. What are the codes for a patient with chronic PTSD? F43.12

14. What are the codes for a patient who has an IQ of 65?   F70

15. What are the codes for a patient with acute exacerbation of chronic myeloid leukemia? C92.10

NERVOUS QUIZ 7

1. What are the codes for a patient with a classic migraine with aura? G43.109

2. What are the codes for a patient with an IQ of 45 who has ringworm? F71, B35.9

3. What are the codes for a patient who has MS? G35

4. What are the codes for a patient who has pars planitis? H30.23

5. What are the codes for a patient who has double vision? H53.2

6. What are the codes for a patient who has pigmentary open-angle glaucoma? H40.1390

7. What are the codes for a patient who has Fusarium keratitis? B48.8, H16.8

8. What are the codes for a patient who has tonic-clonic epilepsy? G40.309

9. What are the codes for a patient who has restless leg syndrome? G25.81

10. What are the codes for a patient who presents today because she has not been taking her insulin as prescribed for her for the past four years and she is now experiencing polyneuropathy due to Type 2 diabetes? E11.40, Z79.4

11. What are the codes for a patient who has presenile cortical cataract of the left eye and is Type I diabetic? H26.019, E109

12. What are the codes for a patient who has epilepsy marked by grand mal seizures which is not responding to treatment? G40.311

13. What are the codes for a patient who has tic douloureux? G50.0

14. What are the codes for a patient who has pseudocyesis? F45.8

15. What are the codes for a patient who has Huntington's dementia? G10, F02.80

TEST 1 ANSWERS

1.   What are the codes for a patient with senile dementia? Z16.30
2.   What are the codes for a patient who has sickle cell anemia Hb-SS with acute chest syndrome? D57.00, J99
3.   What is hemolysis? BREAKDOWN OF BLOOD
4.   What are the codes for a patient who is diagnosed with anemia due to a chronic gastric ulcer? K25.7, D63.8
15.   What are the codes for a patient with benign CKD stage 4 and ASCVD due to hypertension? I13.10, N18.4, I50.9
16.   What are the codes for a pregnant woman who has had three previous miscarriages at approximately 18 weeks and presents today at 20 weeks gestation who is experiencing cramping? O26.22, R10.9
17.   What are the codes for a patient with Crohn's disease? K50.90
18.   What is the term for painful menstruation? DYSMENOHRRHEA
19.   What are the codes for a patient with oophoritis and salpingitis? K50.90
20.   What are the codes for a patient with cellulitis with possible sepsis and COPD with diabetes? L03.90, J44.9, E11.9
21.   What are the codes for a 2-month-old baby who presents with a diaper rash? L22
22.   What is the code for a patient with gastritis after ingesting Percodan with alcohol and OTC antihistamines? K29.60, T40.2X1A, T5.191XA, T45.0X1A
13.   What is the code for a patient with scar tissue due to a second and third degree burn on both legs six months ago? L90.5, T24.009S
14.   What are the codes for an anemic patient due to hemorrhaging of a lower leg wound caused by a car accident? S81.829A, D62, V49.9XXA
15.   What are the codes for a patient with a stage 2 ulcer of the ankle that developed from a cast that was applied to their left lower tibia for 3 months due to a transverse fracture of the shaft? L89.522, S82.225
16.   What are the codes for a patient who has pyogenic arthritis of the hip due to staph? M00.059
17.   What are the codes for a patient with acute and chronic pericarditis? I30.9, I31.8
18.   What are the codes for a patient with amebic carditis? I51.89, A06.89
19.   What are the codes for a patient who has right heart failure? I50.9
20.   What are dilated, swollen, painful veins in the anus or rectum known as? HEMORRHOID
21.   What are the codes for a patient with COPD and emphysema? J44, J43.9
22.   What are the codes for a Type II diabetic patient with neuropathy and pneumonia due to MRSA and a fever? J15.21, E11.40
23.   What are the codes for a patient with asthma that was precipitated by exercise? J45.990
24.   What are the codes for a patient with a perforated appendix with an abscess? K35.3
25.   What are the codes for a patient with RAD? 493.90 REACTIVE AIRWAY DISEASE
26.   What three things must occur for a woman to be diagnosed as having preeclampsia? ELEVATED BLOOD PRESSURE, EXCESSIVE PROTEIN IN THE BLOOD AND EDEMA

27.   What are the codes for a 36-year-old pregnant woman who has a C section due to fetal distress at 39 weeks? O68, O09.513, Z37.0

28.   What is another term for delivery? PARTURITION

29.   What is considered a high blood pressure? 140/90

30.   What are the codes for a patient who has mitral valve stenosis with aortic valve insufficiency? I08.0

31.   What are the codes for a patient who was diagnosed nine weeks ago with chronic coronary insufficiency? I25.9

32.   What are the codes for a 25-year-old pregnant woman who is 33-weeks gestation, has gestational diabetes and is seen today for dehydration? O24.419, E86.0

33.   What are the codes for an 18-year-old pregnant woman who has difficulty in labor due to the birth of a 12 pound baby boy? O65.4, O33.5XX0, Z37.0

34.   What are the codes for a pregnant woman who delivered liveborn twins with one normal and the other breech at 32 weeks with both weighing 5 pounds? O30.003, O32.1XX, O60.14X0, Z37.0

35.   What are the codes for a patient with ASHD and chest pain due to an MI that was treated 10 weeks ago? I25.9

36.   What are the codes for a patient with second degree sunburn? L5.51

37.   What are the codes for a patient with pilonidal cyst with abscess? L05.01

38.   What are the codes for a patient experiencing septic shock due to UTI? N39.0, R65.21303

39.   What are the codes for a patient with goat's milk anemia? D52.0

40.   What are the codes for a patient who metastatic cancer of the uterus? C79.82

41.   What are the codes for a patient who has nonunion fracture of the left humerus? S49.002S

42.   What are the codes for a patient who has degenerative joint disease of the knee? M17.9

43.   What are the codes for a patient who is seen today for a high fever and chest congestion due to the common cold? J00

44.   What are the codes for a patient who has right heart failure?   I50.9

45.   What are the codes for a patient who is diagnosed with pneumothorax due to gunshot wound? S27.0XXA

46.   What are the codes for a patient who has old bucket tear of the lateral meniscus? M23.202

47.   What are the codes for a newborn who was born with a hemangioma of the neck? Z38.00, D18.01

48.   What are the codes when a 1750 gm baby at 28 weeks gestation is delivered due to hypertonic labor? Z38.00, , P03.6, P07.31

49.   What are the codes for a neonate who is diagnosed with diabetes? P70.2

50.   What are the codes for a baby born at 43 weeks who experienced asphyxia due to the cord wrapped around her neck? Z38.00, P84, P02.5, P08.22

51.   What is the code for the newborn when her mother dies during childbirth? Z38.00, P01.6

52.   What are the codes for a patient with second and third degree burns covering 25% of her body with 10% being third degree with infection? T31.21, T79.8XXA

53.   What causes essential hypertension? CAUSE UNKNOWN

54.   What is reactive airway disease? ASTHMA

55.   What are the codes for a patient with lower respiratory infection? J22

56.   What are the codes for an asthmatic patient with status asthmaticus and COPD? J44.0
57.   What is the code for a patient with dislocation of an artificial hip joint? T84.029A
58.   What is the code for a patient with CMV infection due to transplanted liver? B25.9, T86.40
59.   What is the code for a patient with anoxic brain damage resulting from their bypass graft surgery for an MI? G97.81, G93.1
60.   What is the code for a patient with failure of the battery of the pacemaker after two years requiring replacement? T82.111A

CIRCULATORY QUIZ 8

1. What are the codes for a patient with congestive heart failure and hypertension? I50.9, I10

2. What are the codes for a patient with elevated blood pressure? R03.0

3. What are the codes for a patient with malignant hypertensive stage IV CKD? I12.9, N18.4

4. What are the codes for a patient with benign CKD stage 4 and ASCVD due to hypertension? I13.10, N18.4, I50.9

5. What are the codes for a patient with acute and chronic pericarditis? I30.9, I31.8

6. What are the codes for a patient who has a complete AV heart block? I44.2

7. What are the codes for a patient who has strangulated internal hemorrhoids with bleeding? K64.8

8. What are the codes for a patient who has hemiplegia after experiencing a CVA 6 months ago? I69.959

9. What are the codes for a patient who was diagnosed nine weeks ago with chronic coronary insufficiency? I25.9

10. What are the codes for a patient who had an appendectomy due to appendicitis who has postoperative hypertension? I973

11. What are the codes for a patient who is not presenting with any symptoms but was diagnosed as having MI on an EKG reading? I25.2

12. What are the codes for a patient diagnosed with intermediate coronary syndrome? I20.0

13. What are the codes for a patient with chest pain due to acute MI of the inferoposterior wall as part of initial care?   I21.11

14. What are the codes for a patient with RBBB? I45.10

15. What are the codes for a patient who has aplastic anemia due to radiation therapy? D61.1, Y84.2

RESPIRATORY 9

1. What are the codes for a patient with lower respiratory infection? J22

2. What are the codes for an asthmatic patient with status asthmaticus and COPD? J44.0

3. What are the codes for a patient with COPD and emphysema? J44, J43.9

4. What are the codes for a patient with chronic respiratory failure and chronic edema? J96.10, J81.1

5. What are the codes for a patient with ARDS? J80

6. What are the codes for a patient who is dehydrated and has pneumonia of the right lobe? J18.9

7. What are the codes for a patient with pleurisy due to TB? A15.6

8. What are the codes for a collapsed lung? J98.19

9. What are the codes for a patient with a sore throat? J02.9

10. What are the codes for a patient with tonsillitis and adenoiditis? J03.90

11. What are the codes for a patient who is seen today for a high fever and chest congestion due to the common cold? J00

12. What are the codes for a patient with COPD with pneumonia? J44.9, J18.9

13. What are the codes for a patient with acute and chronic bronchitis and COPD? J42, J44

14. What are the codes for a patient with chronic bronchitis and emphysema? J42, J43.0

15. What are the codes for a patient with asthma that was precipitated by exercise? J45.990

DIGESTIVE QUIZ 10

1. What is the code for a patient diagnosed with a peptic ulcer? K27.9

2. What are the codes for a patient with a perforated appendix with an abscess? K35.3

3. What are the codes for a patient with Crohn's disease? K50.90

4. What are the codes for a patient with gastritis and duodenitis? K29.90

5. What is the code for GERD? K21.9

6. What are the codes for a patient with hemorrhagic alcoholic gastritis? K29.21

7. What are the codes for a patient with dysentery and gastritis due to Salmonella? A02.0

8. What are the codes for a patient with Crohn's disease of large and small intestines? K50.80

9. What are the codes for a patient with acute cholecystitis with bile duct calculus and obstruction? K80.43

10. What are the codes for a patient with volvulus with hernia of the intestine with gangrene? K46.1

11. What are the codes for a patient with postoperative hernia? K43.2

12. What are the codes for a patient with acute gastric ulcer? K25.3

13. What are the codes for a patient with gastritis due to alcoholism? K29.20

14. What are the codes for a patient with retropharyngeal abscess? J39.0

15. What are the codes for a patient with incarcerated inguinal hernia? K40.30

INTEGUMENTARY QUIZ 11

1) What are the codes for a patient with severe dermatitis due to her use of pierced earrings? L24.81

2) What are the codes for a patient with infected corn on the right big toe with cellulitis with possible sepsis and COPD with diabetes? L84, J44.9, E11.9

3) What are the codes for a 2-month-old baby who presents with a diaper rash? L22

4) What are the codes for a patient with nonbullous erythema multiforme? L51.0

5) What are the codes for a patient with second degree sunburn? L55.1

6) What are the codes for a patient with exfoliation on 34% of their body due to erythema multiforme with arthropathy? L51.9, L49.3, M12.80

7) What are the codes for a patient with pilonidal cyst with abscess? L05.01

8) What are the codes for a patient with cheloid scar after an appendectomy? L91.0

9) What are the codes for a patient with impetiginous dermatitis? L01.00

10) What are the codes for a patient with impetigo simplex? L01.00

11) What are the codes for a patient with albinism? E70.30

12) What are the codes for a patient with winter's itch? L29.8

13) What are the codes for a patient with dermatitis due to allergy to dust? J30.89

14) What are the codes for a patient with a stage 2 ulcer that developed from a cast that was applied to their right lower leg for 3 months due to a fracture? L89.92

15) What are the codes for a patient with chronic lymphangitis due to staph? B95.8, I89.1

MUSCULOSKELETAL QUIZ 12

16) What are the codes for a patient who has traumatic asphyxiation? S27.9XXA

17) What are the codes for a patient who has pathological fracture of the vertebra due to osteoporosis? M81.0, M80.08XA

18) What are the codes for a patient who has SLE with chronic nephritis? M32.10, N08

19) What are the codes for a patient who has Achilles tenosynovitis? M66.369

20) What are the codes for a patient who has pyogenic arthritis of the hip due to staph? M00.059

21) What are the codes for a patient who has nonunion nondisplaced neck fracture of the left radius? S52.125K

22) What are the codes for a patient who has degenerative joint disease of the knee? M17.9

23) What are the codes for a patient who has chronic obstructive asthma and neuropathy due to Type 2 diabetes which required treatment with insulin because it was uncontrolled? E11.42, J44.9

24) What are the codes for a patient who has old bucket tear of the lateral meniscus of the right knee? M23.200

25) What are the codes for a patient who has a bone spur? M25.70

26) What are the codes for a patient who has acute osteomyelitis of the right ankle and foot? M86.271

27) What are the codes for a patient who has osteopathy due to typhoid fever? A01.00, M90.80

28) What are the codes for a patient who has rheumatic polyarthritis with myopathy? M06.9, G73.7

29) What are the codes for a patient who has carpal tunnel syndrome of the left arm? G56.02

30) What are the codes for a patient who has Sjogren's disease? M35.00

GENITOURINARY QUIZ 13

1. What are the codes for a patient with acute pyelonephritis due to E. coli? N10, B96.20

2. What are the codes for a patient with oophoritis and salpingitis? N70.93

3. What are the codes for a patient with chronic uremia with acute pericarditis? N18.9, N18.9

4. What are the codes for a patient with urinary incontinence and genital prolapse? N81.9, R32

5. What are the codes for a patient with orchitis and epididymitis due to diphtheria? A36.89, N51

6. What are the codes for a patient with menorrhagia? N92.0

7. What are the codes for a patient with post-hysterectomy vaginal prolapse? N99.3

8. What are the codes for a patient with acute cholecystitis with bile duct calculus with obstruction? K80.43

9. What are the codes for a patient with subacute nonsuppurative nephritis? N04.9

10. What are the codes for a patient with renal disease with membranous proliferative glomerulonephritis? N02.2

11. What are the codes for a patient with diverticulitis of the ileum with hemorrhage and peritonitis? K57.13, K65.9

12. What are the codes for a patient with vesicoureteral reflux with bilateral reflux nephropathy? N13.722

13. What are the codes for a patient with ureteral calculus and renal calculus? N20.0, N20.1

14. What are the codes for a patient with posttraumatic renal failure? T79.5XXA

15. What are the codes for a patient with septic UTI due to E. coli? N39.0, B96.20, A41.9

PREGNANCY QUIZ 14

1) What are the codes for a 36-year-old pregnant woman who has a C section due to fetal distress at 39 weeks? O68, Z37.0

2) What are the codes for a 25-year-old pregnant woman who is 33-weeks gestation, has gestational diabetes and is seen today for dehydration? O24.419, E86.0

3) What are the codes for an 18-year-old pregnant woman who has difficulty in labor due to the birth of a 12 pound baby boy? O65.4, O33.5XX0, Z37.0

4) What are the codes for a pregnant woman who delivered liveborn twins with one normal and the other breech at 32 weeks with both weighing 5 pounds? O30.003, O32.1XX0, O60.14X0, Z37.0

5) What are the codes for a pregnant woman who has had three previous miscarriages at approximately 18 weeks and presents today at 20 weeks gestation who is experiencing cramping? O26.22, R10.9

6) What are the codes for a 39-year-old pregnant woman whose baby at 32-weeks gestation is known to have Down's syndrome? O35.1XX0, O09.513

7) What are the codes for a pregnant 23-year-old woman who delivered by C-section a liveborn today at 35 weeks due to severe eclampsia and decreased fetal movement? O15.1, O36.8130, O60.14X0, Z37.0

8) What are the codes for a pregnant woman who delivered a liveborn girl which required an episiotomy to aid in delivery? O80, Z37.0

9) What are the codes for a pregnant woman who delivered twins with a normal delivery? O30.003, Z37.2

10) What are the codes for a 25-year-old pregnant woman who delivered a 10 pound baby boy but the mother's pelvic was too small and forceps had to be used but when these did not work a C-section was done? O65.4, O66.5, O33.4XX0, Z37.0

11) What are the codes for a 38-year-old pregnant woman, 37 weeks gestation, who is seen today for her checkup? O09.51

12) What are the codes for a pregnant 31-year-old woman who is seen today for deep thrombophlebitis which she developed four days after her delivery of liveborn at 42 weeks? O87.1

13) What are the codes for a pregnant woman who had an induced abortion two days ago and

is admitted for a severe infection? O071, Z37.0

14) What are the codes for a pregnant woman who was in a car accident and fractured her tibia? S82.201A, V22.2

15) What are the codes for a woman who delivered a liveborn vaginally at 39 weeks and who had a C-section for her previous pregnancy? O34.21, Z37.0

PERINATAL QUIZ 15

1) What is the code for a liveborn whose was delivered with the use of forceps at 34 weeks and weighing 1260 grams due to placentia previa? Z38.00, P03.2, P07.37, P07.15, P02.0

2) What are the codes for a newborn whose mother was addicted to cocaine and the newborn is experiencing withdrawal? Z38.00, P96.1, P04.41

3) What are the codes for a newborn at this visit who is diagnosed with neutropenia which is not transient? Z38.00, D70.0

4) What are the codes for a newborn with jaundice who was delivered at 34 weeks? Z38.00, P07.37, P59.0

5) What are the codes for a 1-year-old girl who was diagnosed with sepsis due to UTI due to E. coli? A41.50, N39.0

6) What are the neonatal codes for congenital TB?   P37.0

7) What are the codes for a neonate who is diagnosed with diabetes? P70.2

8) What are the codes for a neonate with hyperbilirubinema who was premature at birth and so remained in the hospital with this her third day and weighed 2100 gm at birth? Z38.00, P590, J01.40

9) What are the codes for a baby born at 43 weeks who experienced asphyxia due to the cord wrapped around her neck? Z38.00, P84, P02.5, P08.22

10) What is the code for the newborn when her mother dies during childbirth? Z38.00, P01.6

11) What are the codes for a patient with a bunion on the right foot?   M20.10

12) What are the codes for a 1-month old baby who has not gained any weight? R62.51

13) What are the codes for a patient with lower respiratory infection? J22

14) What are the codes for a fetus whose mother has been diagnosed with rubella? P00.2

15) What are the codes for a newborn whose mother received an anesthetic during delivery with a C-section performed because the newborn's heart rate slowed and was in fetal distress due to the cord being wrapped about her neck with newborn suffering hypoxia? Z38.1, P03.4, P04.0, P02.5, P19.1

CONGENITAL QUIZ 16

1) What are the codes for a newborn who was born with a hemangioma of the neck? Z38.00, D18.01

2) What are the codes for a patient with lateral epicondylitis due to crushing injury? S57.80XA, M77.10

3) What are the codes for a fetus at 35 weeks gestation who is diagnosed with a myelocele and spina bifida of C2-4 and hydrocephalus? Q05.0

4) What are the codes for a newborn during this visit with congenital toxoplasmosis with hydrocephalus? Z38.00, P37.1

5) What are the codes for a fetus who has been diagnosed with Tetralogy of Fallot? Q21.3

6) What are the codes for a missed abortion before 22 weeks for the mother? O02.1

7) What are the codes for an 8-year-old who is seen today for clubfoot that has developed over time? M21.549

8) What are the codes for a pregnant woma n whose baby has been diagnosed with Down's Syndrome? O35.1XX0

9) What are the codes for a 3-day old baby who remains in the hospital after birth due to a diagnosis of Fallot's triad? Z38.00, Q22.2

10) What are the codes for a 30-week pregnant woman with aplastic anemia? O99.013, D61.9

11) What at the codes for a patient who has traumatic asphyxiation? S27.9XXA

12) What are the codes for a 44-year-old man who has arthritis of his shoulder due to Lyme disease? A69.20, M01.X19

13) What are the codes for a 2-year-old child who has been diagnosed with congential hypothyroidism? E00.9

14) What are the codes for a baby born on this visit via C-section with fetal alcohol syndrome due to her mother's alcoholism and occasional cocaine? Z38.01, Q86.0, P04.41

23. What are the codes when a 1750 gm baby at 28 weeks gestation is delivered due to hypertonic labor? Z38.00, , P03.6, P07.31

SYMPTOMS QUIZ 17

1) What are the codes for a 4-year-old patient with high fever, sore throat, and runny nose who is found to have acute right otitis media with rhinitis? J00, H66.90

2) What are the codes for a patient with pathological fracture of the distal radius and COPD with Type I diabetes? M84.439A, J44.9, E10.9

3) What are the codes for a patient who is 82-years-old and broke her right hip and has been severely depressed since? S72.009A, F43.21

4) What are the codes for a patient with second and third degree burns covering 25% of her body with 10% being third degree with infection? T31.21, T79.8XXA

5) What are the codes for a pregnant patient who ws seen for vaginal bleeding at 20 weeks gestation and she had three prior spontaneous abortions at this same time in the pregnancy? O20.9, O26.22

6) What are the codes for a patient who underwent chemotherapy today for small cell carcinoma lung cancer and is now experiencing vomiting without nausea? Z51.11, C34.90, R11.11

24. What are the codes for a patient who has old bucket tear of the lateral meniscus? M23.202

7) What are the codes for a patient with an infected wound of the right humerus which was greenstick fractured with a dislocation and laceration of the axillary nerves? S42.312D, T79.8XXA, S44.31XA

8) What are the codes for a patient with stage 5 renal disease and hypertension as well as arteriolar nephritis and chronic hypertensive uremia? I12.0, N18.5

9) What are the codes for a 45-year-old man with shortness of breath? R06.02

10) What are the codes for a patient with scar tissue of his chest from a third degree burn six months ago? L90.5, T21.31

11) What are the codes for a patient with complaints of dyspnea and tachycardia which the physician believes might be ARDS? R06.00, R00.0

12) What are the codes for a patient with acute and chronic bronchitis with COPD and ASHD? J42, J44, I25.10

13) What are the codes for a 72-year-old man who is seen for elevated liver function studies but hepatitis profile and sugar levels were normal? He is also diabetic Type 2 and has

cholelithiasis. E11.9, K80.20, R94.5, R79.89

14) What are the codes for a 57-year-old man who was admitted to the hospital for possible MI with complaints of chest pain with numbness of the left arm? EKG and stress tests were performed but were negative. R07.9, R20.1

INJURIES QUIZ 18

1) What are the codes for a patient who is diagnosed with pneumothorax due to gunshot wound? S27.0XXA

2) What are the codes for a patient who is diagnosed with a laceration of the right patella with dislocation? S83.091A

3) What are the codes for a patient who is diagnosed with a third degree burn of the chest area? T21.31XA

4) What are the codes for a patient who is diagnosed with comminuted fracture of the shaft of the left humerus with dislocation? S42.351A

5) What are the codes for a patient who is diagnosed with pneumothorax due to stab wound in the chest? S27.0XXA

6) What are the codes for a patient who is diagnosed with swelling of right thumb due to a non-venomous spider bite? S60.361A

7) What are the codes for a patient who is diagnosed with a sprain of the lateral medial collateral ligament of the right knee? S93.411A

8) What are the codes for a patient who is diagnosed with swelling and fever due to rattlesnake bite on her right ankle? T63011A

9) What are the codes for a patient who is diagnosed with second degree burns of the upper right arm? T22.211A

10) What are the codes for a patient who is diagnosed with a pathological fracture of the femur? M84.459A

11) What are the codes for a patient who is diagnosed with frostbite with necrosis of the right ear? T34.011

12) What are the codes for a patient who is diagnosed with a sprain of the posterior cruciate ligament of the left knee? S83.522

13) What are the codes for a patient who is diagnosed with crushing injury of the left lower leg and foot? S87.82XA, S97.82XA

14) What are the codes for a small child who was seen for a bean in his right ear? T16.1XXA

LATE EFFECTS/POISONINGS QUIZ 19

1) What is the code for a patient with an embolism due to their pacemaker?
   T82.817A

2) What is the code for a patient with gastritis after ingesting Percodan with alcohol and OTC antihistamines? K29.60, T40.2X1A, T5.191XA, T45.0X1A

3) What is the code for a patient with scar tissue due to a second and third degree burn on both legs six months ago? L90.5, T24.009S

4) What is the code for a patient with dislocation of an artificial hip joint? T84.029A

5) What is the code for a patient with CMV infection due to transplanted liver? B25.9, T86.40

6) What is the code for a patient with joint pain of the knees from rickets a year ago? M25.561, M25.562, E64.3

7) What is the code for a patient with a pressure ulcer with necrosis from her cast of the left lower leg due to a fractured upper tibia? L97.223, S89.002

8) What is the code for a patient with esophageal reflux due to ingestion of drain cleaner as an attempted suicide? K21.9, T54.3X2A

9) What is the code for a patient with failure of skin graft of the left upper arm sustained after a burn six months ago when boiling water fell on her? T86.821, T22.00XS

10) What is the code for a right-handed patient with hemiparesis of the left side due to a CVA four months ago? I69.954

11) What is the code for a patient with mental retardation due to viral encephalitis more than 5 years ago? F79, B94.1

12) What is the code for a patient with ataxia due to alcohol and carbamazepine? R27.0, T51.91XA, T42.1X1A

13) What is the code for a patient with an infection and pain due to his peritoneal dialysis catheter? T85.71XA, T82.848A, R52

14) What is the code for a patient with sequelae from a gunshot wound of the right leg a month ago? S81.809S

15) What is the code for a patient with dihescence of a mastectomy wound a week ago with infection? T81.32XA, T81.4XXA

SUPPLEMENTARY CODES QUIZ 20

1) What are the codes for a patient seen for follow-up exam of breast cancer which was removed a year ago and treated with chemotherapy? Z08, Z85.3

2) What are the codes for a patient seen who had a replacement of their colostomy? Z43.3

3) What are the codes for a patient seen today for prophylactic administration of Nolvadex for breast cancer which metastasized from skin cancer on the back which was removed a year ago with positive estrogen receptor status? Z79.810, C79.8, Z17.0

4) What are the codes for a woman who delivered a newborn who was 550 grams at 34 weeks with hyperbilirubinemia? O60.14X0, Z37.0

5) What are the codes for a patient who is leaving the country and needed a cholera vaccination? Z23

6) What are the codes for a patient seen today for counseling regarding instructions in the use of an insulin pump for her diabetes Type I and high blood pressure? E10.9, R03.0, Z46.81

7) What are the codes for a patient seen today for cataracts and diabetic neuropathy Type II with long term use of insulin and ASHD? H26.9, E11.40, I25.10, Z79.4

8) What are the codes for a 3-year-old child during a well check who was to receive DTP vaccination but was uncontrollable and so the vaccine was not administered? Z00.129, Z28.89

9) What are the codes for a patient who was seen today for laparoscopic resection of the small intestine with anastomosis which had to be changed to an open procedure for cancer? C17.9

10) What are the codes for a patient seen today for routine PAP test with no findings? Z01.419

11) What are the codes for a patient who is a bone marrow donor? Z52.3

12) What are the codes for a patient seen today for adjustment of peritoneal dialysis catheter during dialysis? Z49.02

13) What are the codes for a patient seen today for possible gout due to complaints of stomach pain but tests were negative? R10.9, Z13.0

14) What are the codes for a patient seen today for exercise therapy after suffering a severe crushing injury to the left lower leg four months ago? Z51.89, S87.80XS

15) What are the codes for a patient seen today for drug resistant pulmonary TB? A15.0, Z16.30

ICD-10   TEST 2

1. What is the code for a patient who is seen today for chest pains due to possible MI? R07.9

2. What is the code for a patient who is seen today for crushing chest injury?   S28.0

3. What are the codes for a patient who has metastatic brain cancer?   C79.31

4. What are the codes for a patient seen today for chemotherapy for ongoing treatment of breast cancer on the right side which was excised two months ago? Z51.11 C50.911

5. An 8-year-old patient is seen today for enteritis due to Clostridium difficile. What are the codes? A04.7

6. What are the codes for a patient who classical PKU? E70.0

7. What does HIPAA stand for? HEALTH INSURANCE PORTABILITY AND ACCOUNTABILITY ACT

8. What other prosecutory actions are levied besides fines for healthcare fraud? PRISON TIME AND CAN'T PROVIDE CARE TO GOVERNMENT PATIENTS

9. What number most often represents an unspecified code? 9

10. What is Volume 2 of the ICD book known as? ALPHABETICAL INDEX

11. Internal derangement of ligament of the left knee is what code? M23.8X2

12. What are the codes for a subsequent encounter for perforation of the esophagus that was traumatic? S27.819D

13. What are the codes for a patient who has cancer of the anterior surface of the epiglottis? C10.1

14. What is the code for postviral encephalitis? A86

15. What are the two supplementary classifications in Volume 1? V AND E CODES

16. Name and describe the three types of health record formats. SOURCE-ORIENTED (BASED ON SPECIALTY OR DEPARTMENT), INTEGRATED (CHRONOLOGICALLY), PROBLEM-ORIENTED (DIAGNOSIS/PROBLEM)

17. Describe the two types of progress notes. SOAP (SUBJECTIVE, OBJECTIVE, ASSESSMENT, PLAN) AND SNOCAMP (SUBJECTIVE, NATURE OF PRESENTING PROBLEM, OBJECTIVE, COUNSELING/COORDINATION OF CARE, ASSESSMENT, MEDICAL DECISION MAKING AND PLAN

18. What does CPC mean? CERTIFIED PROFESSIONAL CODER

19. What types of coding does a CPC perform? PHYSICIAN

20. What are the codes for a patient who has obstetrical tetanus? A34

21. What types of coding does a CCS perform? INPATIENT AND OUTPATIENT HOSPITAL

22. Explain the Stark Laws.   PROVIDERS CANNOT RECOMMEND PATIENTS TO RECEIVE SERVICES FROM AN ORGANIZATION IN WHICH THEY MAY RECEIVE MONETARY BENEFITS

23. What are the codes for traumatic asphyxiation? S71.9XXA
24. What are the codes for a patient who has polio due to having received the vaccine? A80.0
25. What are the codes for benign leiomyoma of the abdomen? D21.4
26. What are the codes for a patient with Reye's syndrome due to when the patient overdosed on aspirin? T39.012, G93.7
27. What are the codes for an intoxicated patient who was binge drinking over the weekend and was seen in the emergency room who experienced alcoholic stupor with blood level of 42? F10.120 R40.1 Y90.2
28. A patient is seen today for arthropathy due to TB in the left shoulder. What are the codes? A18.02 M01.X12
29. ICD-10-CM stands for what? INTERNATIONAL CLASSIFICATION OF DISEASES – 10TH REVISION – CLINICAL MODIFICATION
30. What federal department is CMS a part of? HEALTH AND HUMAN SERVICES
31. How many volumes are there in the ICD today? 3
32. What are the codes for a patient seen today for septic urinary tract infection due to E. coli? A41.51 N39.0
33. What are the codes for a patient seen with hepatitis D associated with inactive Hepatitis B? B17.0
34. What are the codes for a 42-year-old patient who has ASHD in the right leg with gangrene and an ulcer with necrosis where a nonautologous bypass graft was previously inserted? I70.561, L98.493
35. What are the codes for a patient with uveitis due to syphilis? A51.43
36. What is the code for a patient with acute and subacute bronchitis due to Pseudomonas J20.8 B96.5
37. What are the codes for malaria with pernicious complications with hepatitis? B52.8 K75.9
38. What are the codes for a patient who has encephalitis from a tick bite? A84.9
39. What are the codes for a patient who has arthritis of the left hand due to staph infection. M00.042
40. What are the codes for a 23-year-old patient who is seen today for MRSA? B95.62
41. What are the codes for leiomyoma of the uterus? D25.9
42. What are the codes for a patient who is seen today for nausea and vomiting due to chemotherapy? Z51.11 R11.2 C80.1 T88.7
43. What are the codes for a patient with carcinoma of the breast metastatic to the left lung? C50.919 C78.02
44. AHIMA stands for what? AMERICAN HEALTH INFORMATION MANAGEMENT ASSOCIATION
45. What does CCS-P mean? CERTIFIED CODING SPECIALIST – PHYSICIAN
46. What are the codes for patient experiencing panic attack with agoraphobia? F40.01

47. What are the codes for a patient who has MS? G35

48. What are the codes for a patient who has pars planitis? H20.9

49. What are the codes for a patient who is experiencing combat fatigue? F43.0

50. What are the codes for a left snapping knee? M23.8X9

51. A patient is seen today for a stomach ache and headache and was found to be due to pathogenic E. coli food poisoning. What are the codes? A04.0

52. What age is typically defined as presenile dementia.   YOUNGER THAN 65

53. What are the codes for a patient with anorexia? R63.0

54. What are the codes for a patient who has dermatitis due to contact with chromium? L23.0

55. What are the codes for a patient suffering from depression and grief due to the death of her husband? F43.21

56. Describe the CNS.   BRAIN AND SPINAL CORD

57. What are the codes for a patient who has juvenile scoliosis in the cervicothoracic area of unknown cause? M41.113

58. What are the codes for a patient with a classic migraine that is not responding to treatment? G43.119

59. What are the codes for a patient who has spina bifida occulta? Q76.0

60. What are the codes for a patient who has meningitis due to Aerobacter aerogenes? G00.8

61. What are the codes for a patient who has double vision? H53.2

62. What is the difference between hemiplegia and hemiparesis? HEMIPLEGIA IS TOTALLY PARALYSIS ON ONE SIDE OF THE BODY, HEMIPARESIS IS WEAKNESS ON ONE SIDE OF THE BODY

63. Infantile cerebral palsy occurs when? DURING BIRTH

64. What are the codes for a patient who has Fusarium keratitis? B48.8 H16.8

65. What are the codes for a patient who has moderate malnutrition due to low intake of protein? E44.0

66. What are the codes for a patient who has osteitis with chronic mastoiditis due to TB? A18.03 M90.88

67. What does idiopathic mean? NO KNOWN CAUSE

68. When two major changes were added in the ninth revision? EXPANDED FOR HOSPITAL PROCEDURES AND INTRODUCTION OF FIFTH CHARACTER

69. What are the codes for septicemia due to anthrax? A22.7

70. What are the codes for a patient who has erythema multiforme major with inflammation of the eyelid? L51.9, H01.8

71. What are the codes for a pregnant patient who has pneumonia due to anesthesia with aspiration? O29

72. What are the codes for a patient who has Huntington's dementia? G10

73. What are the codes for perforation of the esophagus? K22.3

74. What is the difference between a TIA and a CVA? CVA IS CEREBROVASCULAR DISEASE AND TIA IS TRANSIENT ISCHEMIC ATTACK SO TIA IS TEMPORARY INTERRUPTION OF BLOOD FLOW WITH NO DAMAGE IN CONTRAST TO CVA WHICH CAN BE LONG-LASTING AND DOES PRODUCE DAMAGE

75. What are the fines for healthcare fraud? $10,000 PLUS TIMES 3 PER INCIDENT

OTHER BOOKS BY DR. LYN OLSEN

AVAILABLE NOW AT AMAZON.COM

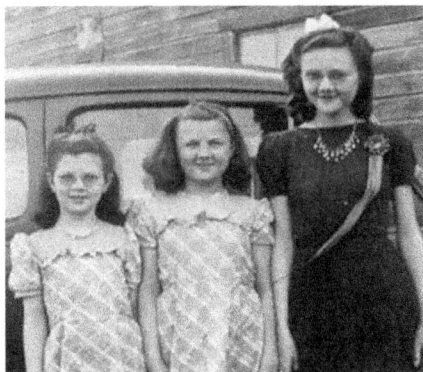

THE THREE SISTERS TRIED AND TRUE RECIPES OF BUTTE MONTANA

DR. LYN OLSEN

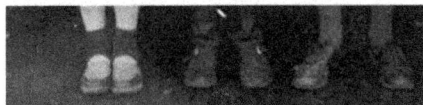

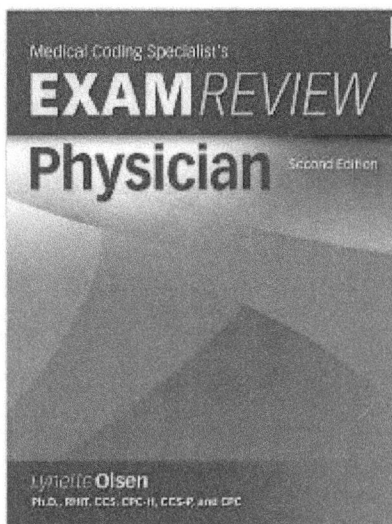

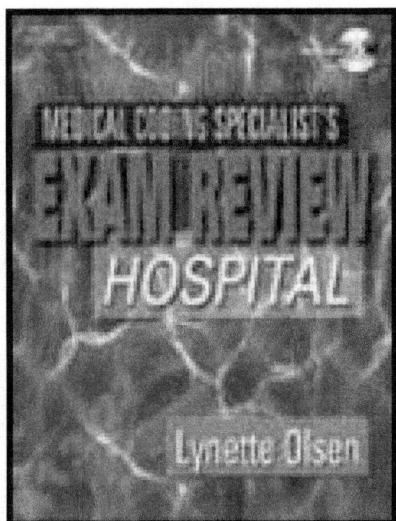

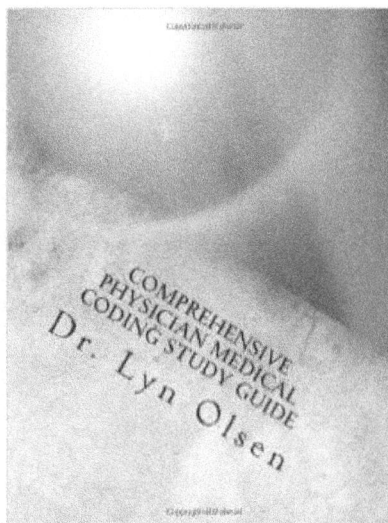

www.ingramcontent.com/pod-product-compliance
Lightning Source LLC
Chambersburg PA
CBHW051209200326
41519CB00025B/7053